Active Living Among Older Adults

Active Living Among Older Adults:
Health Benefits and Outcomes

Edited by
Sandra O'Brien Cousins, Ed.D.
University of Alberta

Tammy Horne, Ph.D.
WellQuest Consulting Ltd.

USA	Publishing Office:	BRUNNER/MAZEL
		A member of the Taylor & Francis Group
		325 Chestnut Street
		Philadelphia, PA 19106
		Tel: (215) 625-8900
		Fax: (215) 625-2940
	Distribution Center:	BRUNNER/MAZEL
		A member of the Taylor & Francis Group
		47 Runway Road
		Levitttown, PA 19057
		Tel: (215) 269-0400
		Fax: (215) 269-0363
UK		BRUNNER/MAZEL
		A member of the Taylor & Francis Group
		1 Gunpowder Square
		London EC4A 3DE
		Tel: +44 171 583 0490
		Fax: +44 171 583 0581

ACTIVE LIVING AMONG OLDER ADULTS: Health Benefits and Outcomes

1 2 3 4 5 6 7 8 9 0

Printed by Edwards Brothers, Ann Arbor, MI, 1998.

A CIP catalog record for this book is available from the British Library.
♾ The paper in this publication meets the requirements of the ANSI Standard Z39.48-1984 (Permanence of Paper).

Library of Congress Cataloging-in-Publication Data
O'Brien Cousins, Sandra.
    Active living among older adults: health benefits & outcomes / Sandra O'Brien Cousins and Tammy Horne, editors.
        p. cm.
    Includes bibliographical references.
    ISBN 1-56032-585-2 (case: alk. paper)
    ISBN 1-56032-817-7 (paper: alk. paper)
    1. Aged–Health and hygiene. 2. Physical fitness for the aged. I. Horne, Tammy. II. Title.
    RA564.8.O267   1997
    613'.0438–dc21   97-38963
                                                                            CIP

ISBN 1-56032-585-2 (case)
ISBN 1-56032-817-7 (paper)

*To the thousands of older adults
who participated in the hundreds of studies
documented here—through you, we learn.*

Contents

Contributors

The chapters in this text represent a team effort and therefore author contributions are not credited by chapter. The list of contributors to the overall effort appears below.

Sandra O'Brien Cousins, Ed.D. (Principal Investigator)[1]
Gordon Bell, Ph.D. (Co-investigator)
Karen Branigan, B.P.E. (Research Assistant)
Art Burgess, Ph.D. (Consultant)
Troy Clamp, B.A. (Research Assistant)
John Cushing, B.A. (Research Assistant)
Vicki Harber, Ph.D. (Co-investigator)
Lorrie Horne, B.P.E. (Research Assistant)
Tammy Horne, Ph.D. (Co-investigator)[2]
Ineke Vergeer, Ph.D. (Co-investigator)
Leonard M. Wankel, Ph.D. (Consultant)

[1] Faculty of Physical Education and Recreation, The University of Alberta, Edmonton, AB, T6G 2H9 Canada.
[2] WellQuest Consulting Ltd., 11511 125 St., Edmonton, AB, T5M 0N3 Canada.

Acknowledgments

This book was made possible by the initiative and financial support of Health Canada's Fitness Directorate through the Canadian Fitness and Lifestyle Research Institute. Specific direction for the work originated with Barbara Shropshire and the Active Living Coordinating Centre for Older Adults (ALCCOA), in preparation for a national consensus conference held in Fredericton, New Brunswick in April 1995. Dean Art Quinney and Dr. Trevor Slack of the Faculty of Physical Education and Recreation of the University of Alberta assisted with the contracting of community research consultant Dr. Tammy Horne and graduate student Sandra Van Vlack to assist in the final stages. Student contributors were Jennifer Glasgow, Chrissy Lengyel, Jill McGuire, Jody Schroh, and Lauri Stratichuk. In addition, the University of Alberta provided computer support, library support, office assistance, and consulting. Appreciation is extended to Doug Zutz and other computer support staff for configuring the department computers so that the bibliographic database could be accessed from two independent computers. In the later stages of the project, Carmen Bassett spent many days making editorial improvements to the material. Makoto and Miho Chogahara spent many hours proofreading and matching references. The editorial comments of Dr. Len Wankel were greatly appreciated.

The team members participating in this project made an enormous effort in identifying, retrieving, reading, and analyzing hundreds of research articles. At times, researchers were pressed to understand and articulate technical information in areas outside their own areas of expertise. Moreover, researchers must be commended for spending many challenging hours, well beyond the original time frame set out in the initial proposal. We hope that the time spent is evident in this book and that the work makes a worthy contribution toward a better understanding of the prospects for better aging through physically active lifestyles.

Chapter 1

Introduction

OVERVIEW OF AGING AND PHYSICAL ACTIVITY

The health and well-being benefits of physical fitness, exercise, and physically active lifestyles have been the subject of a great deal of research in recent years. A number of social trends help to explain the current research interest, across a number of disciplines, in the relationships among aging, exercise, and health: population aging, the wellness movement, increasing leisure time, and concern for rising health care costs.

In North America, there is interest in consolidating knowledge concerning the benefits of, and access to, active living for seniors (Novak, 1994). The concept of active living is similar to that of habitual physical activity. By definition it encompasses leisure-time physical activity, exercise, sports, occupational work, and some types of house and yard work (Bouchard, 1994). Habitual body movement produced by the skeletal muscles and resulting in an increase in energy expenditure can contribute to increased fitness and health.

Orban (1994) advocated that optimal active living should include vigorous physical activity challenges throughout the day to have a full impact on one's quality of life. In this way, reserve energy capacity of the human body adapts to the needs imposed on it.

> Decline in energy capacity with age is a normal phenomenon; abstinence from physical activity is not. Unless one aspires to and embraces a vigorous active lifestyle that includes a habitual supplemental dosage of leisure or occupational physical activity, one increases the risk of impairment, frailty, and morbidity along with a shorter life. (Orban, 1994, p. 161)

Exercise physiologists agree that regular exercise is essential for optimal function of the human body, no matter what the age (Astrand, 1986). Enough evidence exists to prompt Heart and Stroke Foundations in both Canada and the United States to identify physical *inactivity* as a fourth major *modifiable* risk factor for cardiovascular disease, along with smoking, high blood pressure, and high blood cholesterol (Mummery, 1994). The Heart and Stroke Foundations of the United States and Canada acknowledge that research findings are sufficient to recommend that individuals of all ages should be active on a daily basis, because "active is not only basic, it is essential" (Taylor, 1995). Quoting the *Archives of Family Medicine* (1994), Taylor reported, "if just one out of ten U.S. adults began a regular walking program, $5.6 billion in medical care would be saved annually" (Taylor, 1995, p. 2).

The concern for physical inactivity by national health associations is both symbolic and substantial. The Canadian Heart and Stroke Foundation's intent is to alert the public and health professionals that being sedentary exposes individuals to higher risk of death or disability (Taylor, 1993). Russ Kisby, head of *ParticipACTION*, stated:

> It appears that the whole field of preventive medicine is going to be increasingly a priority and fitness/active living fits beautifully right in the middle of that. (Taylor, 1993, p. 3)

There is strong evidence that physical activity reduces the risk of heart disease, and that sedentary people are about twice as likely to develop ischemic heart disease as those who are physically active (Powell, Thompson, Caspersen, & Kendrick, 1987). Economist Louise Wood (1993) estimated that the number of adults with ischemic heart disease would be 16 percent lower and the health care savings about $350 million in one year alone had Canadians' participation in physical activity been twice as high in 1981.

The greatest health benefits from increased physical activity occur when very sedentary persons begin a regular program of moderate aerobic and muscular endurance exercise (Taylor, 1996). Along with the relatively consistent evidence for the physiological benefits of increased activity, there are less consistent findings on the psychosocial and quality of life outcomes related to late-life physical activity such as expanded social networks, reduced depression, and enhanced self-esteem.

Not surprisingly, contemporary research is beginning to address the importance of active living for older people with the notion that achieving an optimal life-span is pointless without satisfactory levels of biological, social, and mental health. North American researchers have been among the first to identify these benefits and to develop understanding about the complex relationships of active living, aging, and health. Ultimately, social policy for health care practice will be affected (and is currently being affected in both the United States and Canada) as it becomes clear just what role active living can play in maintaining independent and healthier living for its aging citizens.

The Active Living Situation of Older Adults

For the purpose of this study, "active living" is defined as "a way of life in which physical activity is valued and integrated into daily life" (Fitness Canada, 1991, p. 4). Active living encourages people to be active in a way that suits their schedules, personal interests, needs, and abilities. Thus a wide array of physical activity was within the scope of this study: formal exercise programs, leisure-time pursuits such as walking and dancing, and recreational and competitive sport participation and domestic activity such as gardening, housework, and paid physical labor.

While physical activity levels are improving, a majority of older people are inadequately active to maintain or improve their health. About half of Canadian seniors reported exercising daily or frequently (National Advisory Council on Aging, 1994). However, in the same study, 36 percent said they *never* exercised. Men at all ages reported significantly more hours per week of moderate, hard, and very hard activity compared to women, and were more involved and capable in vigorous physical tasks which require upper body strength and more strenuous types of movement. Women tended to have better joint mobility. Individuals with less education were more likely to be sedentary. It is not clear how much exercise behavior and capabilities are affected by work, leisure, and gender roles.

Statistics Canada (1992) reported that along with reading, watching television and visiting with family and friends, walking is a frequent activity for noninstitutionalized Canadians over age 65. In the 65 to 69 age group, over half declared that they walk frequently. But by age 75, only 45 percent of seniors reported walking frequently; by age 80, only 35 percent walked. Interestingly, 70 percent of the very old (80+) described their daily physical activity to be already adequate, while only 20 percent admitted that their physical activity was "too little." Clearly, perceptions of daily need for activity is very low in our most elderly citizens.

Among institutionalized seniors in Canada (24 percent of all aged adults), there is no information readily available on daily physical activity patterns. Seventy-two percent of seniors residing in institutions in 1991 were women, and over 40 percent of all women over age 85 can expect to be institutionalized (National Advisory Council on Aging, 1993). Dementia is not the only explanation why so many aged women are institutionalized. Aged women, more than aged men, are more likely to be widowed with no prospect for at-home care following a bout with illness which leaves them weak and frail.

Few care services are currently using physical activity programming as a potential route to restoring muscle strength, bone strength, mobility, balance, and ultimately improved prospects for independent community living. Many older adults may thus succumb to permanent dependency from what could have been a temporary encounter with illness.

However, United States data show an encouraging trend away from sedentary lifestyles among adults ages 65 and over. Between 1987 and 1991, the percentage of the older adult population who reported little or no physical activity declined from 43 percent to 29 percent (U.S. Department of Health and Human Services [USDHHS], 1993).

PROCEDURE FOR THE PRESENT REVIEW

The purpose of this review was to critically examine current and recent research literature regarding the health impact of active living among older adults, assess the state of the evidence for various outcomes, summarize and present the findings, and identify needed and promising directions for future study.

Focus and Limitations

Research has been accumulating from dozens of journals about the importance of physical fitness, exercise, and physical activity for health and longevity. Over 200 journals across a number of disciplines now publish research on the outcomes of physical activity for older adults. This means that, to understand the effects of active living among aging adults, one must survey the literature across a broad spectrum of fields: physical and health education, gerontology, medicine, epidemiology, nursing, physical therapy and rehabilitation, leisure and sport studies, women's studies, health psychology, and medical sociology.

To assess the impact of regular physical activity and active living in later life, longitudinal studies that extended through age 70 and beyond were a priority. Since active living was defined for this project by the Canadian Fitness and Lifestyle Research Institute (1994) as *a way of life in which physical activity is valued as an essential part of daily living*, studies assessing physical activity as part of daily living were given priority. Thus studies which examined short- and long-term outcomes of walking, gardening, domestic physical activity, employment activity, and physical recreative/sport activity were high priority.

However, there were relatively few such studies identified in our searches. The majority of abstracts identified in the CD-ROM searches were not related to the broader active living theme. Active living, as it is practiced in homes and communities, is not well researched. Rather most of the literature utilized pre-post designs on convenience samples, or randomized-control studies using formal exercise. This review thus focused on studies which dealt with the more narrow and conventional definitions of active living, namely, structured physical activity, exercise, and sport.

The most challenging goal of this report was to summarize the evidence regarding active living outcomes (positive and negative) from this vast literature. In addition, we intended to identify areas worthy of further inquiry, but which at present are deficient in quality and/or quantity of information.

This report embodies much of the scientific literature from 1990 to 1994: little literature prior to 1990 is included. Although the study was inclusive of adults ages 50 and older, our work placed a priority on more elderly populations. Particular attention was given to research which explored the consequences of active living in the 70 and older population, since this was where most morbidity and mortality outcomes were likely to become evident.

The vast majority of the literature regarding physical activity outcomes was quantitative and has been generated within the conventional scientific (positivist) paradigm. Qualitative research (e.g., grounded theory, ethnography, phenomenology) was not excluded from the review, but very little research using alternative paradigms (e.g., interpretive) and methods existed regarding physical activity outcomes for older adults. Thus the evidence reviewed in this book is mainly comprised of scientific studies using experimental and correlational research designs and quantitative statistical analysis.

A major limitation of our review was the time frame. The project funding agreement required the review to be conducted within a limited time frame. By the end of the 8-month study, about 1,500 articles had been catalogued representing over 200 journals. Most of these articles were published since 1990 and were selected from approximately 10,000 abstracts. Formal and scientifically controlled intervention studies were the norm. Many studies examined predictors, rather than outcomes, of physical activity. Some articles pertained to other uses of the term "active living" (e.g., getting out and doing sedentary recreational activities with friends). Still, the 1,500 articles we did find are a good representation of the available knowledge available from many disciplines and in many countries.

Production of the Database

To accomplish the task of critically reviewing the literature on active living outcomes among older adults, a number of steps were undertaken. A research team

was developed with a number of investigators and assistants working simultane-
ously on key sections of the study. The research team members were drawn from
a number of the important disciplines needed to address the diverse scientific literature.

Three full-time academic staff of the Department of Physical Education and
Sport Studies at the University of Alberta acted as co-investigators responsible for
supervising aspects of the data gathering and writing and editing section themes.
A community-based research consultant was contracted to co-manage the project.
A recent Ph.D. graduate assisted with the writing, translation, and analysis of the
international literature. Four Master's-level graduate students comprised the data
gathering team, each responsible for surveying primary journals and assisting with
writing. About 20 journals and four specific theme areas were assigned to each
research assistant. Research team meetings were held every week to facilitate
information sharing, problem solving, group decision making, and integration and
joint ownership of the project.

The library system at the University of Alberta is among the best in Canada.
The CD-ROM searches using MEDLINE, PSYCHINFO, SOCIOFILE, and
SPORTDISCUS were very fruitful. Each database explored distinct sets of journals allowing thousands of research abstracts to be found. Keywords appropriate
to each database were used to target the search at adults over age 50 relative to active living and health outcomes. Examples of keywords used were "older adults,"
"aged," "aging," "elderly," "gerontology," "life cycle" *and* "activities," "exercise,"
"aerobic," "fitness," "energy expenditure," "exertion," "leisure time," "lifestyle,"
"outdoor recreation," *and* outcomes such as "longevity," "mortality," "health," and
"life expectancy."

The CD-ROM searches were saved to files on disks which were then reviewed.
A typical CD-ROM file contained several hundred abstracts which were individually screened for their relevance to the project. Abstracts which dealt with active living, health, or performance outcomes and older adult populations were
printed and entered into the PAPYRUS data base (version 7.02) using the *Publication Manual of the American Psychological Association* (1994). In addition,
each study was given an identification number so that it could eventually be stored
in numerical order in a filing cabinet. Up to 10 keywords were also entered with
each scientific article or abstract.

During the writing stage of the project, PAPYRUS keyword searches were
conducted and printed so that research team members could retrieve all the studies
pertaining to a specific theme. Complete articles were then located and analyzed
if relevant. After completing each of their sections, writers returned abstracts and
articles to a locked filing cabinet so that others could access the materials for

their outcome themes, as many of the research studies assessed more than one outcome.

For research areas with a substantial body of literature, team members constructed tables of data for each type of outcome they reviewed. The tables facilitated documentation of the key elements of each study and standardized the way information was collected and presented. The tables laid the foundation for the textual discussion of the outcomes and general evaluation of the evidence.

To assist in critiquing the state of the evidence, the Research Evidence Rating System of Anderson and O'Donnell (1994) was adopted as published in the *American Journal of Health Promotion*. This system was developed to rate scientific studies using quantitative methods. One adaptation was made to this rating system; a sixth category of evidence, "inconclusive" was added. The rating categories and descriptions are:

1. **Conclusive**: Cause-effect relationship between intervention and outcome supported by substantial number of well-designed studies with randomized control groups. Nearly universal agreement by experts in the field regarding impact.
2. **Acceptable**: Cause-effect relationship supported by well-designed studies with randomized control groups. Agreement by majority of experts in the field regarding impact.
3. **Indicative**: Relationship supported by substantial number of well-designed studies, but few or no studies with randomized control groups. Majority of experts in the field believe that relationship is causal based on existing body of evidence, but view it as tentative because of lack of randomized studies and potential alternative explanations.
4. **Suggestive**: Multiple studies consistent with relationship, but no well-designed studies with randomized control groups. Majority of experts in the field believe that causal impact is consistent with knowledge in related areas, but see support as limited and acknowledge plausible alternative explanations.
5. **Weak**: Research evidence supporting relationship is fragmentary, nonexperimental, and/or poorly operationalized. Majority of experts in the field believe causal impact is plausible but no more so than alternative explanations.
6. **Inconclusive**: Research evidence is contradictory. A number of studies with satisfactory designs exist but the findings are not consistent. Further research is needed to clarify the specific conditions under which the findings hold.

SUMMARY OF RESEARCH FINDINGS AND RECOMMENDATIONS

This book presents the findings of an intensive 8-month review and critical evaluation of the scientific evidence concerning health outcomes of active living among older adults, conducted by a 10-member research team at the University of Alberta in 1994. Over 1,500 scientific articles (from over 200 research journals) on various themes relevant to older adults and active living outcomes were identified using keyword searches of CD-ROM databases such as MEDLINE and PSYCHINFO. Articles containing information on adults over age 50, physical activity, exercise or sport, and health or performance outcomes were documented in a bibliographic database. The focus was on the published literature from 1990 to 1994, to keep the scope of the review manageable.

The quantity and quality of scientific evidence related to each theme— physical fitness and health outcomes, specific disease prevention and management, psychosocial well-being outcomes, lifestyle behavioral outcomes, and economic impact—were assessed using a research evidence rating system designed by Anderson & O'Donnell (1994). Added to their five ratings of **conclusive**, **acceptable**, **indicative**, **suggestive** and **weak** was our own category of **inconclusive**. See Table 1-1 for a summary evidence rating for each topical theme.

RECOMMENDATIONS FOR FUTURE RESEARCH

Physical Health and Fitness Outcomes

Of the five thematic sections, physical fitness and performance outcomes are the most rigorously researched. Many topics within this overall theme therefore warrant evidence ratings of "acceptable" or "conclusive." However, a number of topics still require additional study. For instance, research into balance promotion and falls prevention could benefit from standardized assessment tools. Increased aerobic fitness, muscular strength, and joint range of motion are clear outcomes of more physically active lifestyles. Research is needed into the specific nature of programs which help older adults achieve these outcomes. There is much less evidence for outcomes such as obesity reduction, lipid and lipoprotein profile change, and injury outcomes of various physical activities, exercise, and sport.

Table 1-1
Research Themes and Evidence Ratings

Outcome	Rating label[1]
Physical fitness and health	
Cardiorespiratory fitness	Acceptable
Musculoskeletal adaptations	Acceptable
Joint mobility	Conclusive
Body composition	Acceptable
Lipid profile	Weak
Obesity	Weak
Hypertension reduction	Acceptable
Cognitive performance	Indicative
Balance promotion	Acceptable
Falls prevention	Indicative
Injury risk	Suggestive
Specific disease prevention and management	
Alzheimer's disease, dementias	Weak
Coronary heart disease	Acceptable
Bone health	Acceptable
Arthritis	Indicative
Chronic obstructive pulmonary disease	Weak
Cancer	Indicative
Diabetes	Indicative
Mortality outcome	Indicative
Male	Indicative
Female	Suggestive
Sudden death	Acceptable
Psychosocial well-being outcomes	
Anxiety	Inconclusive
Depression	Weak
Self-esteem	Inconclusive
Body image	
Female	Suggestive
Male	Weak
Locus of control	Weak
Life satisfaction	Weak
Knowledge, beliefs, attitudes	Weak
Self-efficacy	
Female	Suggestive
Male	Weak

(Continued)

Table 1-1
(*Continued*)

Outcome	Rating label[1]
Lifestyle behavior outcomes	
Habitual activity level	Indicative
Smoking cessation	Weak
Medication use	Weak
Alcohol consumption	Weak
Nutritional outcomes	Weak
Stress and coping	Weak
Activities of daily living	Suggestive
Economic impact	Weak

[1] Research evidence rating system on Anderson and O'Donnell (1994, p. 7).

Disease Prevention and Management Outcomes

Rigorous longitudinal studies of the link between physical activity and disease prevention outcomes is relatively recent. Thus though the evidence presented in this book is sparse, other evidence does appear to be rapidly accumulating. The role of physical activity in preventing heart disease and promoting bone health among older adults appears to be strong, whereas the relationship between activity and lung disease needs further study. There are a few studies exploring the role of physical activity for specific cancers, diabetes, and prevalent chronic disorders such as arthritis. The role of daily exercise in moderating Alzheimer's disease and other forms of dementia is an exciting new research direction, though present evidence is weak. Although evidence that suggests that an active lifestyle may prevent premature mortality is accumulating, more studies on longevity and premature mortality outcomes are needed, especially for women.

Psychosocial Well-Being Outcomes

There are a number of challenges in researching psychosocial outcomes of physical activity, such as how to define and assess such outcomes. In addition, problems such as "ceiling effects" in healthy populations can make it difficult for researchers to see changes (e.g., if research subjects have high self-efficacy to begin with, there is little room for improvement). It is also likely that the psychosocial outcomes of physical activity among aging adults are altered by a number of contextual factors, such as cognitive function, physical abilities, and social supports.

Because several psychosocial outcomes may occur together, multivariate designs are needed.

Some researchers have expressed concern about the lack of standard assessment tools for psychosocial factors. Such tools would promote ease of comparison across studies. However, given the diversity among older adults in level of cognitive functioning (particularly among the very old), as well as differences in life experiences (as a result of such characteristics as education, culture, gender, and income), it would be problematic to use standardized tools with populations that are different from those with which the tools were developed.

It should also be noted that almost all of the research in this area has been quantitative. Qualitative approaches would be useful for gaining insight into the meaning of various psychosocial outcomes (e.g., how do older adults define life satisfaction and how does an active lifestyle help them achieve it?).

Lifestyle Behavior Outcomes

There has been insufficient research across health behaviors in older age groups. Most of the evidence is weak, but supportive, in suggesting that active living is accompanied by other health-promoting behaviors (e.g., not smoking, eating a healthy diet). Some adults appear to be aging successfully with adequate levels of physical activity, while others, with similar demographic attributes, have adopted sedentary lifestyles and are aging poorly for that choice. More research is needed into what individual and social factors motivate, support, and reinforce physical activity among older adults, versus what barriers (internal or external) exist that limit participation. A positive finding of this review is that habitual activity over time may be self-reinforcing (evidence rating is "indicative").

Measures of activities of daily living (ADLs) are a form of "functional fitness," and these have received enough attention to suggest that active living maintains physical function. More research attending to the direct influence of active lifestyles on late-life independence would be important, both for the individual's quality of life and the economic impact of active living in terms of health care costs.

Economic Impact

Reduced health care costs could be substantial if aging adults remained functionally independent and in good health in late life. The financial implications of maintaining or increasing active living among older adults need further research. Economic impact research involving physical fitness is being conducted with younger, employed adults for the purpose of enhancing corporate productivity and financial profit, but little economic research has been done with older adult populations.

Economic research is difficult, costly, and requires longitudinal studies. Also, in most cost-benefit research, there are a number of ways of calculating costs. Economic studies need to consider a broad range of health and social costs.

Another question that often arises in economic research is "costs and benefits to whom?" For example, if cost savings in the formal health care system are transferred to community-based agencies and individuals, is there really a saving? Economic research on the benefits of physical activity of older adults would need to examine cost savings of both formal health care and community-level and informal care, and also take into account any costs to older adults themselves of staying active.

Advice to the Reader

The remainder of the report is organized into five major categories of outcomes: physical health and fitness outcomes, disease prevention and management outcomes, psychosocial health and well-being outcomes, lifestyle behavioral outcomes, and economic impact outcomes. Each major category contains a number of outcome theme (topic area) sections which are presented in a standard format. A written section discusses the strengths and weaknesses of the research studies which were found, summarizes key findings, and presents the overall evidence rating for that outcome. Finally, theme sections covering a well-researched outcome conclude with table(s) depicting intervention or comparative research (pre-post intervention studies or comparative studies of active versus inactive groups) and/or correlational or epidemiological research (studies using noncausal multivariate designs).

In the "findings" column of each table of intervention or comparative research, significant relationships are given a (+) if the exercise intervention group was significantly different, at post-test, from a control or comparison group or from a pre-test (for single group repeated measures designs). A (+) **n.s.** indicates a change in the dependent variable which approached, but did not reach, significance. A (−) indicates that there was no relationship found or no change in the dependent variable.

Abbreviations are often used in the tables for brevity. The full meaning of technical abbreviations is given upon the first use of that word or phrase. Because of limited space in the tables, the reader is reminded that the extracted information in the tables is a summary and lacks contextual information. Please refer to the original scientific paper for full understanding.

There will be some variations in style among the many sections of this book because several researchers were involved in the writing. For instance, some of the discussions are more in-depth and describe specific studies, whereas other sections are more general and limit detailed coverage of specific studies to the summary tables. Also, the evidence rating for each section was decided by the researcher who was chiefly responsible for writing that section.

Chapter 2

Physical Health and Fitness Outcomes

CARDIORESPIRATORY FITNESS OUTCOMES

Summary

Overall, the evidence rating for cardiorespiratory outcomes of active living in older adults is **acceptable**. Aging is associated with a reduction in cardiorespiratory fitness resulting in a decline in VO_2max (aerobic fitness) by approximately 10 percent per decade after the age of 25. Previous athleticism and training that is continued throughout life can reduce this relative decline in VO_2max by about 50 percent.

Research has demonstrated that low-, moderate- and high-intensity aerobic exercise training initiated later in life can play a beneficial role in attenuating this decline. In addition, the relative improvements in VO_2max observed after training in elderly males and females are similar and comparable to that seen in healthy younger subjects after exercise training. However, the adaptations that mediate these changes may differ between females and males.

Other assessments of cardiorespiratory fitness such as anaerobic threshold and submaximal endurance variables show similar improvements with physical activity in the elderly. A limitation of the present literature is that there remains a paucity of data assessing the effects of aerobic training or strength training (either alone or in combination) for individuals in their ninth and tenth decades of life. Thus, future research should address the effects of various forms of exercise training in this very old cohort.

Discussion of the Evidence

Cardiorespiratory (CR) fitness involves the ability of the cardiovascular (CV) and respiratory systems to take in and deliver oxygen utilized by the working muscles (Astrand, 1986). The single best assessment of cardiorespiratory fitness has been the maximal oxygen consumption test (VO_2max). Other variables such as anaerobic threshold and submaximal endurance performance have been used. According to the Fick equation, VO_2max is the sum of cardiac output (Q) and arterial oxygen content (the central component) and the peripheral component of arteriovenous oxygen difference (a–VO_2). Controversy exists regarding which component is the "weak link" limiting VO_2max in younger healthy sedentary or athletic individuals (Green & Patla, 1992; Wagner, 1992). Increased age is associated with a decline in cardiovascular structure and function and VO_2max (Robinson, 1938; Dill et al., 1967; Heath et al., 1981; Ogawa et al., 1992).

In healthy sedentary males and females, VO_2max declines by approximately 10 to 14 percent per decade after the age of 25 (Heath et al., 1981; Khort et al., 1991). The decline in VO_2max has been attributed to disease, disuse, or deconditioning associated with a sedentary lifestyle and to age-related changes in cardiovascular structure and function and the atrophy of skeletal muscle. Other cardiorespiratory fitness variables show a similar age-related decline (Inbar et al., 1994). The purpose of this section is to assess the role of physical activity in offsetting the age-related decline in cardiorespiratory fitness.

A physical training investigation by Ogawa et al. (1992) demonstrated that the decline in VO_2max was attributable to both central and peripheral limitations. Nearly half the age-related decline in VO_2max and cardiac output was attributed to a diminished maximal stroke volume while peak heart rate and arteriovenous oxygen difference accounted for the remainder of the decline (Ogawa et al., 1992). The above results contrast to the findings of Rodeheffer et al. (1984) who did not observe a decline in peak stroke volume or cardiac output during exercise. Thomas et al. (1993) suggested that the age-related reduction in cardiovascular response to both light and strenuous exercise may not be as large as previously reported. Therefore at the present time, the precise role that the central and peripheral components play in the observed age-related decline in VO_2max remains somewhat equivocal (not unlike findings for younger people).

Despite the reduction in VO_2max, individuals who continue to train and compete on a regular basis later in life have been shown to attenuate the decline in VO_2max by approximately 5 percent per decade, thereby cutting the age decline in half (Kasch et al., 1990; Aoyagi & Katsuta, 1990; Rogers et al., 1990). Based on the above observation, other studies have investigated the role of aerobic exercise training, in previously sedentary individuals, in offsetting the age-related decline in VO$_2$max (Aoyagi & Katsuta, 1990; Kasch et al., 1990; Kavanagh & Shephard, 1990).

Short-term (4 weeks) or long-term (1 year) aerobic exercise training initiated later in life (at 60 to 80 years) has been shown to increase VO$_2$max by 7 to 38 percent in both male and female subjects (Seals et al., 1984; Blumenthal et al., 1989; Makrides et al., 1990; Belman & Gaesser, 1991; Ehsani et al., 1991; Kohrt et al., 1991; Govindasamy et al., 1992; Hamdorf et al., 1993). Govindasamy et al. (1992) demonstrated that significant improvements in VO$_2$max can occur in as little as two weeks of training in previously sedentary elderly individuals. This improved cardiorespiratory fitness has been attributed to both central and peripheral adaptations including an increase in:

(a) maximal stroke volume (Seals et al., 1984; Ehsani et al., 1991),
(b) ejection fraction and left ventricular contractile function (Ehsani et al., 1991),
(c) cardiac output (Ehsani et al., 1991; Makrides et al., 1991),
(d) arteriovenous oxygen difference (Seals et al., 1984; Frontera et al., 1990), and
(e) maximum ventilation (Seals et al., 1984; Govindasamy et al., 1992).

In addition to improved maximal cardiorespiratory fitness, endurance training also increases the lactate and ventilatory thresholds (Blumenthal et al., 1989; Belman & Gaesser, 1991; Govindasamy et al., 1992; Takeshima et al., 1993) and decreases submaximal endurance performance (submaximal heart rate, endurance time, physical work capacity, and so on) and myocardial oxygen demand (DeVries et al., 1989; Ehsani et al., 1991; Hamdorf et al., 1992, 1993; Keyser et al., 1993; Babcock et al., 1994). Some research has not shown an increase in ventilation threshold with a combined arm and leg endurance training program of 12 weeks despite an increase in peak oxygen uptake and submaximal exercise heart rate (Keyser et al., 1993). Master athletes have been shown to have an enhanced oxidative capacity of skeletal muscle that can increase the peripheral component of cardiorespiratory fitness (Coggan et al., 1990).

In deconditioned sedentary or frail elderly individuals who have reduced muscle volume and muscular strength, it may be possible that an exercise regimen consisting of lower extremity strength training may increase muscle mass, maximal muscular strength, and peak power output, resulting in a significant improvement in cycle ergometer VO$_2$max. Frontera et al. (1989) assessed the effects of high-intensity lower extremity strength training on maximal muscular strength and VO$_2$max in elderly individuals between 60 and 72 years of age. The 3-month strength training routine resulted in a marked improvement in lower extremity muscular strength (107%), muscle fiber area, and citrate synthase activity, resulting in a small (6%) but significant improvement in VO_2max. Therefore, further studies need to assess the role of strength training alone or in combination with aerobic training to offset the age-associated decline in musculoskeletal and cardiorespiratory function.

Males have a greater cardiac output and oxidative capacity of skeletal muscle than females, which produces significantly higher VO_2max and submaximal endurance performance for males (Suominen et al., 1977; McElvaney et al., 1989; Spina et al., 1993). The relative improvements observed in cardiorespiratory fitness are somewhat similar between the genders (Suominen et al., 1977; Cress et al., 1991; Spina et al., 1993; Warren et al., 1993). However, Spina et al. (1993) found that the factors that contribute to the increase in VO_2max may differ. The greatest contributor to the increase in VO_2max was the increase in stroke volume for the males and arteriovenous oxygen difference in the females (Spina et al., 1993).

A limitation of the current literature assessing the effects of exercise training in elderly individuals is the focus on the young old (65 to 75 years), with few controlled studies addressing the effects of exercise training on the middle old (75 to 85 years) or the very old (85 years and older). Because the population is aging and there will be a greater percentage of individuals living well into their ninth decade, it is necessary that future research address the potential role of exercise in enhancing cardiovascular function in this cohort. Also, it is well known that the change in cardiorespiratory fitness is dependent on initial fitness, genetic limitations, and program design (frequency, intensity, duration, and mode of training).

Table 2-1 summarizes intervention or comparison studies concerning cardiovascular fitness outcomes of active living for older adults. No strictly correlational studies were reviewed, given that most of the research in this area involves intervention studies or comparisons among groups (e.g., younger versus older adults, active versus sedentary older adults).

MUSCULAR STRENGTH OUTCOMES

Summary

The overall evidence rating for muscular strength outcomes is **acceptable**. The majority of intervention studies indicate that resistance training results in significant strength gains in the elderly and especially among the frail elderly. Strength

Table 2-1

Cardiorespiratory Fitness Outcomes: Intervention and Comparison Studies

Researchers and sample	Design, treatment, and measures	Findings
Spina et al. (1993); 31 subjects, healthy volunteers, 15 men and 16 women. Mean age = 64 years	Intervention group only. 2 to 3 months flexibility, then endurance training for 9 to 12 months of walking, jogging, rowing, cycling. 45 minutes per session, 5 days per week initially at 60 to 70% of HRmax, then 75 to 85%. Measured VO_2max, a-vO_2 difference cardiac output, stroke volume (SV).	(+) Significant increases in VO_2max, Qmax, Svmax, and a-vO_2 diff. were observed in males but only VO_2max and a-vO_2 diff. was significantly increased in females. Females may increase VO_2max via peripheral mechanisms whereas males increase both central and peripheral aspects of VO_2max with training.
Govindasamy et al. (1992); 12 men. Mean age = 66.5 years	Intervention group only. Jogging or walking, 4 times per week at 70 to 75% VO_2max. Measured VO_2max.	(+) VO_2max increased by 6.6 % after 4 weeks and increased another 5.2% after 5 more weeks of training.
Posner et al. (1992); 247 men & women. 60 to 86 years	Exercise group (randomly assigned) trained 40 min for a total of 16 weeks, 3 times a week at an intensity of 70% peak HR. Control group had lifestyle talks. Measured VO_2max work rate at ventilation threshold (VT).	(+) VO_2max increased 8.5% for exercise group, decreased for control group. Work rate at VT increased by 5% in exercise group and decreased by 8% in controls.
Khort et al. (1991); 53 men and 57 women, healthy and sedentary for 2 years; 60 to 71 years in age	Intervention group only. Walking and jogging for 45 minutes a day for 9 to 12 months, 3 to 7 days per week at 80% of HRR. Measured VO_2max.	(+) Increased VO_2max = 24%; increase in VO_2max independant of age, sex, or initial fitness level.

(Continued)

Table 2-1
(*Continued*)

Researchers and sample	Design, treatment, and measures	Findings
Relman & Gaesser (1991); 18 men and women, 65 to 75 years of age, no CV, bone, or joint disease.	Randomly assigned to high-intensity (HI) or low-intensity (LI) training. Walking 30 min a day for 8 weeks, 4 days a week. LI = 35% HRR, and HI = 75% HRR. Measured VO_2max, Lactate threshold (LT).	(+) VO_2max increased 7% for LI and HI. LT increased 12% for LI and 10% for HI.
Coggan et al. (1990); 8 male Master's athletes (age = 63) competing in endurance events.	Master's athletes compared with comparison group of younger athletes with similar performance times. Measured VO_2max, muscle biopsy data (fiber type, enzymes, capillarization), self-reported training.	VO_2max lower in Master's athletes but no difference in fiber type. Some muscle enzyme activities and capillary to fiber ratios higher in master athletes. Master's athetes also had higher cross-sectional area of type I fibers. Thus, peripheral component to CR fitness in master's athletes was maintained or better than younger athletes with same endurance times.
Makrides et al. (1990); 24 men, 12 were 20 to 30 years; 12 were 60 to 70 years, sedentary, screened for CV or respiratory disorders.	12 interval programs, 3 days a week at 65% to 125% peak VO_2 per hour. VO_2max, cardiac output (Q), a-vO_2 diff.	(+) Young VO_2max increased 29%, Q increased 14%, a-vO_2 diff. increased 14%; older VO_2max increased 38%, Q increased 30%, a-vO_2 diff. increased 6%.

(*Continued*)

Table 2-1

(*Continued*)

Researchers and sample	Design, treatment, and measures	Findings
Hagberg et al. (1989); 57 men and women, 70 to 79 years	Randomly assigned to control, endurance, or resistance group; 3 per week for 26 weeks, endurance training at 50 to 85% VO_2max; resistance training: 8 to 12 reps on 10 Nautilus machines. VO_2, 1Rep maximum.	(+) Endurance training increased VO_2max by 22%; no change in resistance group. Resistance training group increased upper and lower body strength by 18% and 9% respectively.
Seals et al. (1984); 24 men and women, 60 to 69 years	14 exercise subjects; 10 controls 6 months low-intensity (LI) followed by 6 months of high-intensity (HI) training; LI (20 to 30 min walking) 3 times a week for 6 months at HRR 120 bpm; HI (30 to 45 min) at 75 to 85% HRR. Measured VO_2max, Q, a-vO_2 diff., stroke volume (SV), ventilation (Ve)	(+) LI: VO_2max increased 12%, Q no change, a-vO_2 diff. increased by 6%, SV increased by 6%, and Ve also increased; HI: VO_2 increased by 18%, a-vO_2 diff. increased 9%, and Ve increased.
Kasch et al. (1990); Subjects were followed over 18 years. Mean age was 44.6 and 51.6 years before and 68.0 and 69.7 years after the study.	15 exercisers and 15 nonexercisers (exercise dropouts). Measured resting HR and BP, VO_2max	(+) VO_2max declined with age in both groups but significantly more in nonexercisers suggesting that regular exercise retards the age-related loss in aerobic power.

training and regaining lost muscle function caused by decreased activity is important for maintaining independence in the performance of activities of daily living.

Musculoskeletal adaptation to strength training is most rapid during the first 8 weeks of training. Further changes in strength tend to plateau with only small increases observed following 8 weeks. Both type I and II fiber areas increase in response to training and a relationship has been identified between changes in strength and fiber area.

Older adults should be encouraged to involve themselves regularly in resistance forms of exercise that load muscles beyond normal daily requirements. The maintenance of muscle strength above task-dependent levels is important for the easy resumption of tasks needed to continue independent living following a bout of illness.

Concentric and eccentric forms of strength assessment are lacking, compared to isometric types of programs. Since hypertension is so prevalent in the elderly, and in consideration of the fact that daily living is not always isometric in nature, further research is recommended to examine forms of resistance training other than isometric forms.

Studies of greater duration and intensity may illustrate the potential for the elderly to adhere to strength training programs. Additionally, longer-term supervised exercise programs may demonstrate which factors are associated with strength gains including changes in sense of well-being as a result of independence levels in activities of daily living.

Discussion of the Evidence

Advanced age is a significant factor accounting for declines in muscle strength. Total muscle mass decreases as individuals age, with the greatest decrease occurring after 50 years of age. The reduction of muscle mass has been estimated at approximately 33 percent between the ages of 30 and 80 years. This loss accelerates to approximately 1 percent per year after the age of 70 (Heislein et al., 1994; Rantanen et al., 1994).

Other factors are known to contribute to changes in muscle strength and weakness in the elderly. These include postural changes, the accumulation of chronic diseases complicated by medications used to treat them, disuse atrophy (deconditioning), and under-nutrition (Fiatarone & Evans, 1993). Thus the actual decline in strength which can be attributable to age alone is not entirely clear, and some evidence suggests that the decline can be slowed by about 50 percent with formal physical training (Shephard, 1989).

The evidence presented in the contemporary literature indicates that strength-oriented exercise programs lead to highly beneficial outcomes for the elderly population. Even mild activities can lead to improved muscle function while scientifically controlled progressive resistance training can lead to improvements in strength of over 100 percent (Fiatarone et al., 1994). In more frail populations, increased muscle activity can reverse serious functional consequences of sedentary aging which otherwise would result in the reduction in muscle volume, muscle strength, and aerobic capacity (Avlund et al., 1994). McMurdo and Rennie (1994) randomly assigned volunteers of average age 83 to either a seated exercise program or reminiscence therapy. They concluded that physical activity was an important influence in reducing the disablement process in frail elderly.

The recognition that the elderly can benefit from formalized strength training programs has been illustrated by many researchers (e.g., Era et al., 1994; Pyka et al., 1994; Avlund et al., 1994; McMurdo & Rennie, 1994; Heislein et al., 1994; Fiatarone et al., 1994). Researchers have identified benefits associated with strength training in elderly individuals which include increased performance in functional abilities such as activities of daily living (feeding, bathing, dressing, housekeeping, transportation, and moving about without fatigue).

Along with increased muscle strength, psychological parameters such as sense of control, self-esteem, body image, and life satisfaction may be altered, but studies are needed to clarify how the improved muscle function (i.e., strength) is translated into improved mental outlook and better perceptions about one's body.

Although current research has identified that elderly participants can benefit from participating in training to increase muscular strength and in turn quality of life through independent living, further research is needed. Very few of the studies completed have utilized standardized and established means of formalized strength training which ultimately could have even more potent outcomes for the elderly. Standard programs require that a repetition maximum (RM) be determined at the outset so that progressive training can occur based on this initial individualized standard. Without this customized format, individuals are rarely loading their muscles optimally and are likely to make slower progress.

A few studies have attempted to use progressive overload training methods (Fiatarone et al., 1994). Pyka et al. (1994), along with Dupler and Cortes (1993), applied a progressive overload methodology in which the participants completed given sets and repetitions at a percentage of their one-repetition maximum. Other investigations have had subjects perform strengthening exercises including weighted stair climbing (Cress et al., 1991) and the use of elastic bands and body positioning (Heislein et al., 1994) to increase the intensity of exercise.

Measurement of strength in the elderly is often performed utilizing isometric (static) exercises that are known to raise blood pressure. Few studies have utilized isokinetic or isotonic dynamic movements that may be a safer way to evaluate performance. Additionally, many investigators have trained elderly subjects using seated isometric exercises for people who are more frail. Studies utilizing dynamic movement and apparatus such as tubing and light weights may elicit different responses to resistance exercise.

Generally, the sample populations utilized in contemporary research are nonrepresentative of the older adult population as a whole. Sample participants are primarily recruited from medical treatment facilities, old age homes, or rehabilitation centers (Heislein et al., 1994; McMurdo & Rennie, 1994; Fiatarone et al., 1994). A few researchers (Dupler & Cortes, 1993; Cress et al., 1991; Pyka et al., 1994) have recruited volunteer subjects who are fully active in the community and their homes to train in their study. The utilization of active, healthy, and independent elderly subjects requires future research to focus on prevention outcomes rather than rehabilitation benefits.

Increasing or maintaining optimal strength as an outcome of active living needs to be a more important focus of future research. Can everyday activities of daily living including dressing, feeding, domestic activities, and locomotion maintain an individual's strength at an acceptable level? It is not clear whether older individuals can promote or maintain their strength by engaging regularly in everyday at-home activities. Research is needed to determine if resistance activities, conducted in the unsupervised conditions of one's home, can make a difference to functional fitness. Also helpful would be research using tasks equating the strength and endurance contributions of active living events such as 30 minutes of raking or 10 minutes of snow shoveling or digging, to formal resistance program outcomes.

Studies with larger samples of both female and male elderly subjects need to be conducted. Some of the larger studies have evaluated strength as a one-time isometric measure without an intervention (Era et al., 1994; Avlund et al., 1994). Periods of training longer than 8 to 10 weeks would be useful especially if followed by an evaluation of subjects' adherence to the exercise intervention. Resistance training exercise may be difficult without ongoing supervision and we need to know whether independent training or even dependent (supervised) training is sustained in older people as a behavior change. Motivational research suggests that many women are adverse to muscle development at any age; other work suggests that fears regarding over-exertion may be operating (O'Brien Cousins, 1995). Additionally, future researchers need to apply larger load and intensity to determine the ideal intensity and dose-response characterstics for maximal strength increases in elderly subjects.

Table 2-2 contains summaries of intervention or comparative studies. Table 2-3 summarizes correlational or epidemiological studies.

JOINT MOBILITY OUTCOMES

Summary

In general, the level of evidence for joint mobility outcomes is **conclusive** for certain joints in nondiseased adults. Joint flexibility is an important outcome of

Table 2-2
Muscular Strength Outcomes: Intervention Studies

Researchers and sample	Design, treatment, and measures	Findings
Pyka et al. (1994); 25 adults ages 61 to 78 years (avg. 68.2); 8 male, 17 female.	Subjects randomly assigned to exercise or control group. Resistance training for 15, 30, and 50 weeks; 16 subjects in exercise and 6 in control group for 15 and 30 weeks; 8 subjects in exercise and 6 in control group for 50 weeks; 12 resistance exercises involving all major muscle groups. 3 x per week for 1 hour, 3 sets of 8 reps. Measured 1-repetition maximum (RM); number, change in types I and II fibers and fiber area.	(+) Significant increase in strength following 8 weeks of training. Further changes in strength tended to plateau with only small increases for 15 weeks; strength values differed significantly between control and exercise groups.
Heislein et al. (1994); 22 females; aged 50 to 64, patients recruited from two hospitals.	Intervention group only. Progressive weight-bearing sequence; resistance increased with elastic bands. 1 x per week supervised and 2 x per week home sessions for 8 weeks. Measured strength with an isometric dynamometer; quads, hamstrings, grip strength.	(+) 21% increase in quadriceps strength ($p < .001$); 9% increase in hamstring strength ($p < .07$); 14% increase in grip strength ($p < .002$).
McMurdo & Rennie (1994); 65 adults ages 67 to 98 years; avg 83 years.	Subjects were randomly assigned to seated exercise group ($n = 36$) or to the reminiscence therapy group ($n = 29$). 45 min. of seated isometric exercise sessions accompanied by music, or reminiscence therapy encouraging social interaction and group discussions. Two exercise sessions per week at unspecified intensity; two reminiscence sessions per week. Measured quadriceps muscle strength 1RM, step test.	(+) Regular low-intensity seated exercise improved quadriceps strength in the very elderly; supports the trainability of muscles in even the frail elderly. Physical activity reverses the disablement process.

(*Continued*)

Table 2-2
(*Continued*)

Researchers and sample	Design, treatment, and measures	Findings
Fiatarone et al. (1994); 100 adults avg. age 87.1; 63 females, 37 males agreed to participate, residents of the Hebrew Rehabilitation Center of the Aged.	Exercise and nonexercise groups (nonrandom). Resistance training; placebo activities (walking, seated calisthenics, board games, concerts, and group discussions). Measured muscle strength and size, body composition, mobility.	(+) Muscle strength increased 113% in the exercise group and 3% in the non-exercise group ($p < .001$). Gait velocity increased 11.8% in exercise group but declined 1.0% in the non-exercise group ($p = .02$). Stair climbing power increased 28.4% in the exercise group vs. 3.6% in the non-exercise group ($p = .01$). Cross-sectional thigh muscle area increased by 2.7% in the exercise group but declined 1.8% in the non-exercise group ($p = .11$).
Dupler & Cortes (1993); 20 subjects; 11 males, 9 females. Male ave age 69.4, female ave age 62.8. Subjects all active, independent, and completely ambulatory. Free from blood pressure complications and orthopedic problems.	12-week standardized weight training program based on individual's 1RM. 3 days/week of high intensity training (avg 63.5% of 1RM weight training load). Training intensity ranged from 45% of 1RM during week 1 to 75% of 1RM during weeks 11 and 12. Various strength and body composition measures taken.	(+) Female average strength increased 72.2% ($p < .001$). Male average strength increased 66.1% ($p < .00001$). Body composition remained virtually unchanged. Lean body weight increases were not significantly different pre- or post-training.

(*Continued*)

Table 2-2
(*Continued*)

Researchers and sample	Design, treatment, and measures	Findings
Cress et al. (1991); 31 female subjects volunteered, 27 completed the study; 65 to 86 years; avg. age 72.	Measured activity level, VO_2max, strength, muscle biopsy, histochemical analysis; muscle fiber area.	(+) Significantly increased thigh strength, vastus lateralis type IIb fiber area, and VO_2max. Exercise group type IIb fiber area increased by 29%, post-training versus the decline of 22% in the controls.

Table 2-3
Muscular Strength Outcomes: Correlational and Epidemiological Studies

Researchers and sample	Measures	Findings
Avlund et al. (1994); 405 older adults (mean age = 75). Random selection.	Physical activity level; functional ability, maximal isometric strength.	(+) Regular low-intensity seated exercise is positively related to quadriceps strength in the frail elderly. Level of physical activity is related significantly to musculoskeletal function and functional ability.
Era et al. (1994); 541,441, and 382 people (both sexes) from 3 different communities; avg. age = 75; Norwegian elderly.	Maximal isometric strength: hand grip; arm flexion; and knee extension strength; various anthropometric measures; functional tests (10 m. walking speed; stair mounting test).	(+) Significant relationship between strength measures and functional tests. Maintenance of muscle strength above task-dependent levels is important for independent living.

physical activity and should not be underestimated for its essential role in maintaining basic functional fitness. For some elderly people, mobility may be even more important to independent living than aerobic fitness.

The spine, hip, and shoulder joints are key locations of the body where flexibility can be regained. The knee and elbow joints, however, do not gain much mobility. The ankle joint may also be resistant to mobility change. Other joints such as fingers and wrists have not been studied to any extent. In general, frail populations of elderly may need more time to increase their mobility and can expect more modest increases in joint range of motion (ROM).

Discussion of the Evidence

Joint Range Of Motion (ROM) is a physical parameter that people believe naturally declines with age. Many people may think there is little they can do about losses in flexibility. Yet evidence is accumulating that older people can obtain and maintain a great degree of flexibility. Some joints are not susceptible to the same level of physiological losses seen in muscle strength and aerobic fitness. Flexibility of the hip, spine, and shoulder can be improved, while mobility of ankles and knees may be difficult to alter.

Noteworthy about flexibility gain is that immediate improvement of joint mobility may be possible within a single exercise session and this occurrence may increase motivation for older adults. Studies with pre-post measures on a single session of exercise are warranted.

It could be argued that joint flexibility is not a very important fitness component compared to aerobic fitness. However, for the elderly, not being flexible enough to cut toenails, put on socks, connect a brassiere, or do a proper breast self-examination (BSE) is a serious limitation. In fact it could be argued that without adequate joint mobility, independent living is indeed compromised making range of motion an essential health and quality of life consideration.

The only longitudinal study data on range of motion changes of older women who participate in regular exercise was conducted by Misner and colleagues (1992). Following 12 females ages 51 to 71 when the study began, this research team set up a three times per week exercise program of a 15 to 30 minute stretching period followed by 30 to 60 minutes of elective walking or water aerobics. All stretches were done slowly, moving through the range of motion 5 to 10 times, and holding the stretch for 8 to 10 seconds for each repetition. Subjects were tested every 6 months, and at least five times over the 5 years with the Leighton flexometer for assessing shoulder flexion, shoulder extension, shoulder transverse extension, hip flexion, and hip rotation. Except for shoulder flexion, all joint ranges improved significantly. Most improvement occurred in the first 6 months, although hip flexion continued to improve after that period. Misner et al. concluded that "age-related losses in range of motion can be forestalled by a regular program of exercises specifically directed at improving range of motion of joints" (p. 41).

As with strength, joint *specificity* is an issue. The types of movements that are habitual dictate which joints are regularly activated. Therefore lifestyle factors affect the degree of restriction versus mobility that older people experience in joints: people influence their anatomical mobility just by how they live and by what they do. For example, a study on a randomized-control sample of older female volunteers found that nondiseased spinal mobility can be significantly increased in only 10 weeks with a 20- to 30-minute program of gentle stretching three times per week (Rider & Daly, 1991). The interesting aspect of the spinal mobility study is that the control group was also in the same exercise class, but only the experimental group did the spinal mobility exercises. This type of investigation demonstrated that "locomotor forms of exercise, including walking, jogging, dancing, and other forms of movement are not sufficient by themselves in improving one's spinal mobility" (Rider & Daly, 1991, p. 217).

There is some evidence to suggest that "morning stiffness" is a measurable phenomenon which is associated with grip strength and other functional abilities which improve over the course of the day (Ferraz et al., 1992). Thus, researchers warn that in older people, scientific measures of mobility and functional status that are repeated over the course of the study must be taken at the same time of each study day.

An interesting study on BSE in women age 65 and older found that upper extremity mobility was an essential requirement for adequate performance in BSE (Baulch et al., 1992). Limitations and deficits in range of motion of the shoulders and hands were a problem for self-examination. More study is needed to determine the role of range of motion exercise in correcting self-examination disability. The need for research in this area is indicated in order to improve assessment and education of older women regarding the use of proficient BSE for early detection of breast cancer.

BODY COMPOSITION OUTCOMES

Summary

The overall level of evidence for body composition outcomes of active living among older adults is **acceptable**. Advancing age is associated with changes in body composition, including increased fat mass and decreased fat-free mass (FFM). As a percentage of body weight, age changes are from 10% bone, 30%

Table 2-4
Joint Flexibility Outcomes: Intervention and Comparative Studies

Researchers and sample	Design, treatment, and measures	Findings
Mulrow et al. (1994); 163 frail nursing home residents dependent in at least two activities of daily living (ADLs).	Subjects randomly assigned to physical therapy (PT) sessions or friendly visit (FV) control group, 4 months duration. PT included range of motion, strength, balance, transfer, and mobility exercises (session length time N/A). One-on-one therapy exercise or visit time 3x/week. Measured range of motion.	(−) No significant diff. in range of motion. Concluded that a standardized PT program provided little mobility benefits for very frail long-stay nursing home residents.
Bautch (1993); 30 adults living independently with osteoarthritis (OA) of the knee.	2 groups of 15 subjects each randomly assigned to Exercise or Education group. Exercise group: 1 hr. of ROM, walking and joint protection training. Education: 1 hour session on health, exercise, or arthritis education; Exercise 3x/week at < 60% VO_2max; education 1x/week. Measured Arthritis Impact Scale of 45 items, Pain (Visual Analog Scale); Borg Ratings of Perceived Exertion; Walking Ability in metabolic equivalents (METs) using speed and grade on treadmill.	(+) Reduced joint pain and improved mobility. Both groups reported a significant improvement in Functional Ability. The Exercise group reported a significant improvement in level of pain for both "pain now" and "pain in the past week." No change in Work Capacity or Walking Ability.
McMurdo & Rennie (1993); 49 subjects; average age = 87 years; 64 to 91; from 4 seniors, residences in Dundee, Scotland.	Subjects randomly selected. Participated in exercises to music ($N = $ 12F, 3M) or reminiscence activity ($N = $ 21F, 5M). 45-minute sessions; 2 sessions/wk; for 7 mos. Measured goniometer assessment of active knee extension, active knee flexion, spinal flexion.	(+) Significant difference for spinal flexion in exercisers ($p < .00001$); (−) Knee mobility did not improve significantly.

(Continued)

Table 2-4
(*Continued*)

Researchers and sample	Design, treatment, and measures	Findings
Brown & Holloszy (1991); 75 subjects ages 60 to 71 (no age diff. among groups); Non-smokers from St. Louis, MO; in good health and free of orthopedic problems; 64.6 years.	Self-selected to exercise and control groups. 62 exercisers: 30 F, 32 M; 13 controls: 6F, 7M; 60 minutes of general exercises as described on a worksheet (no supervision) 5 days per week for 3 mos. Independently paced exercise (no exercise leader). Goniometer assessment of ankle dorsi and plantar flexion ROM, lying hip flexion, hip extension, forward bending range.	(−) No change in ankle ROM was observed for either group. (+) Significant increases in exercisers flexibility on forward bend, straight leg raise, hip extension, and hip internal rotation. Control group had no significant changes.
Rider & Daly (1991); 20 females; average age 71.8 years; volunteers, medically screened, free from orthopedic problems and osteoporosis and willing to take up flexibility training.	Subjects were all in an exercise class, but randomly assigned to 10 who got special flexibility exercises and 10 control who did not. Exercised 20 to 30 min/day; intervention group did 4 spinal mobility or flexibility exercises including back flexion and extension; 3 to 5 repetitions per session, each held for 10 seconds, 3x/week for 10 wks. (supervised training); spinal flexion (sit and reach); spinal extension while lying (linear distance of chin from floor).	(+) Significant improvement of sit and reach flexion of 28.4 cm to 32.6 cm; spinal extension of 17.9 cm to 25.0 cm. Control group declined on sit and reach .5 cm and increased on spinal extension by 1.2 cm. ANOVA with repeated measures revealed significant spinal mobility improvements in experimental group but not controls even though they were in same exercise class.

(*Continued*)

Table 2-4
(Continued)

Researchers and sample	Design, treatment, and measures	Findings
Hopkins et al. (1990); 65 females; ages 57 to 77; mean age = 65; community-living volunteers.	Subjects randomly assigned to groups (35 exercisers, 30 controls); 50-minute exercise sessions of stretching, walking, and dance movements 3x/week; 12 weeks at target heart rate of 100 to 120 beats per minute (bpm). Flexibility was assessed using the modified Sit and Reach Test.	(+) Significant improvement 28 cm to 30.5 cm (9%) MANCOVA using pre-test measures as covariates indicated significant positive change in sit and reach flexibility; control group had 0% change.
Blumenthal et al. (1989); 101 (51F, 50M) ages 60 to 83; average = 67 years; recruited volunteers through television, magazines, radio, and newspapers; medically screened.	Subjects randomly assigned to aerobic exercise ($N = 33$); yoga & flexibility ($N = 34$); wait list control ($N = 34$); 1 hour of warmup exercise, 30 minutes of cycling, brisk walking/jogging, and arm ergometry, cool-down; 3x/week for 16 weeks with cycling at 70% of maximum heart rate. Assessed perceived improvement (in %) of flexibility.	(+) Significant difference in perceived improvement. The aerobic and yoga exercisers both reported positive changes in their flexibility of 84% and 91% respectively while the control group perceived 0% improvement.

muscle, and 20% adipose tissue in young adults to 8% bone, 15% muscle, and 40% adipose tissue by age 75. Fat mass and fat-free mass have both been independently linked with health outcome.

Both aerobic activity and resistance training can moderate age-related changes to body composition but must be of sufficient duration, frequency, and intensity. The best activities for maintaining bone and muscle mass are those that provide mechanical strain and are weight-bearing.

Data from body composition measurement techniques must be interpreted with caution. Common techniques such as body mass index (BMI) and skinfold measures offer no information about relative fat mass or FFM percentages. Data can be strengthened when used with other valid measures (dual energy X-ray absorp-

Table 2-5
Joint Flexibility Outcomes: Correlational Studies

Researchers and sample	Measures	Findings
Duncan et al. (1993); 39 men; 3 groups based on low, intermediate, and high ability to walk on their own. 69+ years, average age = 75; disease-free at Durham Veterans Hospital.	Groupings were based on walking ability: Low ($N = 16$; unable to descend stairs without a handrail); Intermediate ($N = 10$); High ($N = 13$; can descend stairs without a railing and walk 5 steps without assistance). Assessed goniometer measures of right and left ankle dorsiflexion and plantar-flexion; knee flexion and extension; hip extension (10 variables).	(+) Significant differences between the groups on left knee flexion and right ankle dorsiflexion (ANOVA). Individuals with low walking ability had lower flexibility scores. However causality is not indicated.
Voorrips et al. (1993); $N = 50$; 3 groups based on activity level: active, intermediate, inactive, average age = 71.5 years; door-to-door recruitment; The Netherlands.	3 activity levels (groups) based on a one-time questionnaire of physical activity. Assessed flexibility of hip and spine.	(+) Significant differences between the 3 study groups for flexibility of the hip and spine. Active people are more flexible; causality is not indicated.

tiometry or hydrostatic weighing). Further research is needed to determine age-appropriate measures for elderly women and men.

Discussion of the Evidence

Body fat under the skin decreases with age. Fat becomes internalized in the trunk with age, especially in men, and some women who have a more "android" (male) body shape. Excessive fat mass at the waist is associated with a long list of medical problems, including cardiovascular disease, hypertension, some forms of cancer, and diabetes mellitus. On the other hand, a reduction in fat-free mass is associated with significant loss of muscle strength and capacity as well as loss of bone or osteopenia. The combined result of these age-related changes often deprives the individual of living an independent life and reduces her or his potential for carrying out the daily tasks of living. Minimizing the gain in fat mass and the loss of fat-free mass that occurs with normal aging will provide most individuals the best opportunity to live a high quality life of good health.

There are many body composition measurement techniques, and each has its strengths and limitations. Body mass index (BMI) and skinfold measurements are commonly used to estimate body composition. These results must be interpreted with caution for several reasons. BMI is calculated from a person's body weight and height and offers no insight into body composition. This measure should be used in combination with other data such as a waist-to-hip circumference ratio. Skinfold equations developed in the middle-age population and elderly assume a constant fat-free density. This may lead to an overestimation of body fatness because of the bone mineral loss with age. However, a decrease in the water content of the fat-free mass with age lessens the bone mineral effect. Further work is required on age-appropriate measurement techniques and equations for elderly men and women.

Routine physical activity contributes significantly to positive changes in body composition. There is an inverse relationship between recreational activity and body weight change after 10 years of follow-up. Those subjects who report regular activity over their lives gain less body weight compared to those who self-report little or no regular activity. Aerobic activities (walking, jogging, swimming, cycling) have typically been recommended for minimizing fat mass gains. Participation must exceed 12 weeks at an intensity of at least 50 percent of maximal oxygen consumption for these benefits to be observed.

More recently, resistance exercise has been promoted for preserving fat-free mass. The body composition benefits noted from resistance training are consistently reported in the literature. Several studies note that participation in resistance training programs (3 days/week, lifting weights at 80% of their one-repetition maximum for 16 or more weeks) leads to a reduction in percent body fat and an increase in lean tissue. Muscle strength gains range from 5 percent to 65 percent, depending upon the type of resistance exercise used, the exercise protocol, age of the participant, and baseline strength. The greatest gains are usually observed in those muscle groups that have been under utilized or rarely trained before. Older men and women experience similar improvements relative to each other and to their younger exercising peers.

Other body composition benefits observed from regular activity include the maintenance or remineralization of bone. Bone responds best to weight bearing activity and those activities that provide direct mechanical strain to the bone (i.e., resistance training). Therefore, walking can make a contribution to the leg bone, but not the arm bone.

LIPID AND LIPOPROTEIN PROFILE OUTCOMES

Summary

The level of evidence for blood cholesterol outcomes of active living is **weak and somewhat confusing because of insufficient data**. With advancing age, total cholesterol and triglyceride levels become higher while the effect on high- and low-density lipoproteins is not as clear. Women often have higher levels of high-density lipoprotein (HDL-C) than men without the same health risk. Generally, total cholesterol and HDL-C levels are strong indicators of potential heart disease.

A serum lipid/lipoprotein profile associated with reduced coronary disease is often observed in individuals with a physically active lifestyle. The independent effect of exercise on blood lipid and lipoprotein levels, however, is difficult to detect. Findings from cross-sectional and longitudinal studies often conflict. Also, many studies lack randomized sedentary control groups and confounding variables such as age and gender are not always controlled.

An exercise-induced change in lipid and lipoprotein profile appears to be threshold-dependent and may vary across age levels and between women and men. Exercise at 65 percent of maximal oxygen consumption for 30 minutes, 3 times per week, appears to be beneficial but exercise must be maintained to sustain positive effects.

Discussion of the Evidence

Serum lipids and lipoproteins undergo relatively predictable changes with age. Total cholesterol (T-CHOL) and triglycerides (TGs) are higher with advancing age, but the effects of age on high-density lipoprotein (HDL-C), the "good" cholesterol, and low-density lipoprotein (LDL-C) are not as clear.

The literature is very consistent with respect to the risks associated with particular lipid and lipoprotein profiles. A favorable blood profile would include T-CHOL less than 6.2 mmol/L and an elevated HDL-C:LDL-C ratio. The strongest health link is with heart disease and related heart problems. Coronary heart disease (CHD) is responsible for significant morbidity and mortality in both men and women.

Some gender differences between blood profiles have been reported. The Framingham study reported that serum T-CHOL and HDL-C were independent risk factors for coronary heart disease (CHD) in elderly women and men. Serum TG was an independent risk factor for CHD in elderly women but not men. In persons over 65 with prior myocardial infarction, T-CHOL was most strongly related to CHD and all-cause mortality. Several researchers have noted that patients may have normal T-CHOL but abnormal HDL-C associated with CHD, and thus HDL-C may be a stronger indicator of potential heart disease.

Active people often have favorable plasma lipid/lipoprotein profiles compared to inactive people. A physically active lifestyle is associated with a serum lipid/lipoprotein profile associated with reduced CHD. An active person's profile would likely show a decrease in TG and an increase in HDL-C. In addition, the typical rise in age-related TG is not seen in fit subjects.

The cross-sectional and prospective study results do not always agree. Cross-sectional studies often report an improved HDL-C profile with regular exercise but some prospective randomized control trials do not observe changes in HDL-C with regular exercise of up to 2 years duration. For example, in a cross-sectional study of 1,273 women, Reavan et al. (1990) reported higher HDL-C but similar T-CHOL, LDL-C, and TG levels in elderly women who self-reported regular exercising versus not exercising.

In contrast, following a meta-analytic review of 27 longitudinal studies, Lokey and Tran (1989) concluded that exercise reduces T-CHOL and TG. However, significant changes in HDL-C were generally not observed. Furthermore, when the findings were adjusted for body weight, the change to T-CHOL and TG was not seen.

A critical appraisal of the literature demonstrates that many research studies fail to consider potential confounders such as hormonal status, phase of the menstrual cycle, and body composition. Results from longitudinal studies are often inconsistent and difficult to interpret because of experimental design problems (e.g., inadequate type, duration, intensity of exercise intervention, lipid measurements made across the menstrual cycle [levels vary 10–25% across cycle], and studies carried out in women with a high baseline HDL-C). Most studies have neither used randomized sedentary control groups nor monitored and adjusted for changes in body weight or dietary habits. Consequently, the independent effects of exercise on blood lipid and lipoprotein change are difficult to ascertain.

Lipid/lipoprotein changes appear to be activity threshold-dependent and baseline TG-dependent. A common recommendation is to exercise at 65 percent of maximal oxygen consumption for 30 minutes, at least 3 times per week. In addition, positive results are noted if baseline TG = 1.25 mmol/l (120 mg/dl). Endurance-trained subjects demonstrate a better lipid/lipoprotein profile compared to resistive-trained or sedentary peers who have been matched for body fat. These changes can occur rapidly and are likely caused by an increase in lipoprotein lipase activity with an acute bout of exercise. The exercise regimen must be maintained regularly to sustain the positive effects. HDL-C may be more sensitive to total volume of exercise rather than intensity (1200–1500 kcal/week required for 12 or more weeks). Other researchers suggest that exercise must be maintained at sufficient intensity (60% of maximal heart rate or more) for an increase in HDL-C to be experienced.

Women tend to have higher HDL-C levels than men and subsequently may not be as responsive to exercise. Cross-sectional studies confirm that active women have higher HDL-C levels than sedentary women but intervention studies suggest that training programs (in the absence of other interventions) do not improve HDL-C significantly in older women even though high-intensity exercise in young women does increase HDL-C. This suggests that an exercise-induced change in HDL-C may be threshold-, age-, and gender-dependent and require vigorous exercise. Women may need more activity compared to their male counterparts.

OBESITY OUTCOMES

Summary

The overall evidence rating for obesity outcomes of active living in older adults is **weak**. Aging is associated with an increase in fat mass and a drop in fat-free mass. Exercise reduces fat mass but builds muscle (hypertrophy), sometimes leading to a heavier but leaner body. Approximately 25 percent of men and women between the ages of 20 and 74 years are overweight with fat. Women have a higher probability of gaining fat weight in their adult years.

There are little data on obesity specific to an aging population and the impact of regular physical activity. Remaining physically active seems to help prevent age-related weight gain. Also, physically active overweight adults have lower morbidity and mortality rates than those who are not active.

There is mixed evidence about the effectiveness of exercise for weight loss because fat that is lost may weigh less than the lean muscle gained. Activity by itself increases energy expenditure, but a combination of diet and exercise appears to lead to a greater loss of weight and fat mass than does exercise alone. Inconsistent findings also result from varying experimental design (especially length of exercise trial), poorly matched subjects (e.g., on baseline level of adipose tissue), and inadequacies in recording of dietary intake.

Weight loss appears to be threshold- and adiposity-dependent. Physical activity should be performed at a low to moderate intensity within a range of 50 percent to 75 percent of maximal aerobic capacity to promote fat utilization.

Discussion of the Evidence

Obesity is associated with a lengthy list of medical problems and chronic disease. These include an increased risk of diabetes mellitus, insulin resistance, hypertension, cardiovascular disease, hypertryglyceridemia, decreased levels of HDL-C, increased levels of LDL-C, gallbladder disease, some forms of cancer, sleep apnea, chronic hypoxia, hypercapnia, and degenerative joint disease. For example, the prevalence of hypertension is 2.9 times higher in the obese compared to the non-obese population. Research suggests that one-third of all hypertension cases are caused by obesity.

The definition of obesity varies and is dependent upon the tool used to estimate body fatness. BMI, which is calculated as body weight(kg)/height(m)^2, is the most commonly used index for obesity. By this measure, overweight is defined as a BMI of 27.8 or more in men and 27.3 or more in women. For persons of average height (men 5'9", women 5'4"), the body weight would be equivalent to more than 85 kg for men and more than 72 kg for women. These BMI are also approximately equivalent to 25 percent body fat in men and 32 percent body fat in women. Severe obesity is defined as a BMI of greater than 40 or greater than 35 with medical complications. BMI offers no insight into body composition (i.e., proportion of fat mass to fat-free mass) and therefore should be used in combination with other methods such as bioelectric impedance or waist-to-hip ratio.

Using the above-described BMI definition, among U.S. adults ages 20 to 74 years, 24 percent of men and 27 percent of women are overweight. The severely overweight population is made up of 8 percent of men and 10.6 percent of women.

Women have a higher probability of gaining weight in the adult years. Gender differences in prevalence, duration, and intensity of voluntary weight loss attempts might explain the observed differences in body weight and weight change. Although women have a greater predisposition to weight gain, women must define obesity by health standards, not cultural standards. Many women who are not overweight undertake diets and may subsequently generate weight problems for themselves unnecessarily.

Causes of obesity are not well defined and genetics appear to play a role. A common misconception is that the obese eat too much or are very inactive. This is not necessarily the case. Physical inactivity (or cessation of activity) or excess food intake contribute to development of obesity but are not the only causes. Weight gain is often associated with the individual's initial body weight, smoking cessation, and diuretic medication. Weight gain is negatively associated with baseline physical activity or an increase in activity. Because of regional differences in metabolic activity of fat stores, upper body fat is more readily mobilized compared to lower body fat.

In recent years it has been determined that fat distribution (body type) and duration of obesity are more important risk factors (e.g., for heart disease) compared to total body fat. Visceral or internal fat and central fat (abdominal/chest) are related to disease risk such that a predominant trunk distribution of body fat increases risk of mortality. Heart disease risk increases significantly for a waist-to-hip ratio (cm/cm, or inches/inches) that is greater than 1.0 or greater in men and 0.8 in women.

There are little available data specific to an aging obese population and the impact of regular physical activity. Remaining physically active may help prevent age-related weight gain. In addition, the physically active overweight have lower morbidity and mortality rates, but there are mixed reviews about the effectiveness of exercise and weight loss. Activity, by itself, increases energy expenditure but a combination of diet and exercise appears to lead to a greater loss of weight and fat, as well as an improved waist-to-hip ratio and a healthier lipid/lipoprotein profile when compared to dieting or exercising alone. When exercise and dieting are combined, fat-free mass is preserved and can subsequently increase resting metabolic rate.

The studies that have examined the effect of diet and/or exercise on weight loss in the obese are difficult to interpret, and making generalized statements about these strategies is impossible. The problems associated with most studies are the variable initial levels of obesity of the subjects, the extremely variable length of exercise trials, and lack of dietary tracking or assessment for most subjects.

The effect of exercise on weight loss among obese individuals is not a dose-response relationship. In other words, increasing levels of activity does not ensure predictable or continued weight loss. In several studies conducted with twins, the data describe a large inter-individual variation in the amount of weight change. Weight loss is a product of one's energy balance (i.e., caloric intake and energy expenditure), generating different body composition in each individual and suggesting that weight loss is threshold- and adiposity-dependent.

Most studies indicate that participation in activities that burn less than 200 kcal each day, performed 3 times/week for 12 to 24 weeks leads to little fat loss. The literature recommends that weight loss exercise should be performed within a range of 50 percent to 75 percent of maximal aerobic capacity to promote fat utilization. This level of activity is preferred compared to those of higher intensity. Exercise programs have received some criticism because alone they do not generate as great an energy deficit as food restriction. However, exercise creates and preserves fat-free mass and therefore assists in the maintenance of an ongoing higher metabolic rate.

It is recommended that all obese individuals consult a physician before commencing any exercise program. The moderately obese face minimal risk when

Table 2-6

Body Composition, Nutrition, Obesity, and Lipid Profile: Intervention and Comparative
Studies

Researchers and sample	Design, treatment, and measures	Findings
Butterworth et al. (1993); women ages 72 to 73 years; trained group (65 to 84 years, competitive, trained 1 hour/day for last 5 years, VO_2 max > 26 ml/kg) used for baseline comparison only. Others healthy, 67 to 85 years, no smoking or alcohol abuse, no disease, no diets or exercise programs.	Subjects randomly assigned to walking with HR monitors ($n = 14$) or supervised calisthenic exercise ($n = 12$). Controlled for body weight and diet during study; 7-day food records collected at baseline, 5 wks and 12 wks; 5 days/wk, 30–40 min/day at 60% HRR for 12 weeks; 2 dropouts from walking due to foot injury, 30 of 32 complied with study protocol. Measured body weight, BMI, and skinfolds (sum of 4), VO_2max.	(+) Body weight, BMI, and skinfolds (sum of 4) significantly lower and VO_2max significantly higher in trained vs. other 2 groups. Walking group consumed significantly more energy and nutrients compared to sedentary group. One in walking group vs. up to 10 sedentary below 67% recommended daily allowance (RDA) for several nutrients. Increased VO_2 (12.6%) with walking. (−) No change in body composition or nutrient intake. No association between increased activity and increased quality of dietary intake.
Nieman et al. (1993); see Butterworth study from above, same study.	See Butterworth above.	(+) HDL significantly higher (26%), lower TG (36%) in walkers compared to sedentary group. (−) Similar total cholesterol and LDL between groups. No significant change in lipid profile with 12 weeks of exercise. Cross-sectional data suggest that high levels of physical activity (1.6 hr/day for > 5 years) combined with leanness may have little impact on serum cholesterol and LDL of elderly women but tend to be associated with elevated HDL.

(Continued)

Table 2-6
(*Continued*)

Researchers and sample	Design, treatment, and measures	Findings
Webb et al. (1993); 17 males ages 55 to 77; no CHD, normal ECG, blood pressure (BP), no medications, obesity, or diabetes.	11 exercisers, 6 controls; 8 weeks of endurance cycling; 3 times/wk; 30–60 min/session at 60%–75% VO_2max. Measured resting metabolic rate, body density, VO_2max, sodium – potassium (Na-K) pump.	(+) Increased resting metabolic rate 10% in normotensive men. Decreased blood pressure 5%. (−) No change in body composition. Small sample size, low-intensity program.
Kohrt et al. (1992); 47 males and 46 females ages 60 to 70 years; non-smokers, no meds, no previous exercise, normal BP and rest/exercise ECG.	9 to 12 month aerobic program (walk, jog, row, cycle); 3 to 5 times/wk, 30–50 min/sessions, 60%–85% HRmax (gradual increase). Measured skinfold, VO_2max, fat mass, fat-free mass, BP, blood glucose, lipid profile.	(+) Males skinfold fat drop more at central and upper body sites, females skinfold drop equally at all sites. Training may retard central fat accumulation (which is associated with CHD) but skinfold does not look at internal fat stores. Improvement in blood profile may be linked with change in body composition.
Whitehurst & Menendez (1991); 34 females ages 61 to 81 (average age = 69); normal ECG, BP, no chronic disease, no BP meds, no previous exercise.	20 walking; 14 controls; walking 8 weeks; 3 times/wk at 70%–80% HRmax; 20–40 min/session. Measured HDL. 2 walkers and one control did not complete post-test.	(+) Increased HDL in walkers, though baseline difference in body composition between walkers and controls may explain stronger lipid response in walking group. Lipid response was intensity-dependent.

commencing an exercise program, but those with severe obesity are more resistant to weight loss and are often unable to perform many activities because of sheer size and musculoskeletal problems. Only a few studies have focused on the severely obese. Studies are often too short, and the adherence of the subjects to exercise is extremely low. Some measured biochemical markers have shown small improvements post-exercise while others have shown no change. For example, improved insulin sensitivity and a decrease in resting norepinephrine levels have been documented. Further examination of the type of exercise and its protocol (frequency, intensity, and duration) when combined with controlled dietary intake is required.

HYPERTENSION OUTCOMES

Summary

The overall level of evidence for hypertension outcomes of active living among older adults is **acceptable**. Hypertension, as assessed using direct and indirect blood pressure measures,[1] has been shown to be lower in active elderly subjects compared to the sedentary and obese elderly.

Some controversy exists as to the effectiveness of physical actitivity in reducing hypertension in the elderly and between women and men. However, in sedentary, hypertensive, or obese elderly subjects (regardless of gender) blood pressure can be lowered with physical activity if the exercise stimulus is sufficient in terms of intensity, frequency, and duration and if positive lifestyle and nutritional practices are followed.

Hypotension (low blood pressure) may be a problem for some older individuals and has been associated with falls. Further research is necessary to evaluate the role physical activity may have in reducing orthotic hypotension.

Discussion of the Evidence

Hypertension can be clinically described as chronically increased systemic arterial pressure. Diagnosis of hypertension is made by measuring blood pressure, with 140 mmHg systolic and 90 mmHg diastolic suggested as setting the upper limits. Hypertension may be the result of an increase in cardiac output or total peripheral resistance.

The physiological causes of hypertension include kidney disease or damage (renal hypertension) which produces an increase in renin and subsequent angiotensin II, which elicits vasoconstriction and an increase in systemic pressure. Primary hypertension (approximately 90% of all cases) has been associated with

---

[1] Blood pressure can be measured directly using an indwelling catheter attached to a pressure transducer inserted into an artery, or indirectly using a sphygmomanometer. Indirect blood pressure measurement techniques have been criticized as having a high degree of variablity in measurement and thus limited validity. Significantly lower blood pressure values have been observed with indirect compared to direct techniques (Wiezek et al., 1990). However, indirect measures are common in the literature and research using such measures is included in this review.

Table 2-7
Body Composition, Nutrition, Obesity, and Lipid Profile: Correlational and
Epidemiological Studies

Researchers and sample	Measures	Findings
Aronow & Ahn (1994); Men (259 with coronary artery disease, 288 normals), women (515 CHD, 731 N) 62 years or older. Average age 80–83 ± 8; Chol ≥ 200 mg/dl, HDL ≤ 35 mg/dl CHD = MI, ECG evidence of angina pectoris.	Cross-sectional, single blood sample: total cholesterol, HDL, LDL, TG; CHD.	(+) High total cholesterol and LDL cholesterol, low HDL were risk factors for CHD in elderly men and women; were independent risk factors for CHD. HDL very important regardless of total cholesterol.
Rantanen et al. (1994); 1,388 older adults in sample, 909 in strength test; average age 75 years; from 3 regions of Finland; different participation rates by region (transportation problem; variable medical exams, or subjects felt they were "too healthy").	Cross-sectional data collected only one time; maximal isometric muscle strength (hand, elbow flex, knee ext, trunk ext/flex), medical, anthropometric measures (BMI + BIA), lean body mass.	(+) Lean body mass strongly correlated with absolute isometric strength. Different absolute strength was found among geographic regions, occupation, and previous activity levels.
Danielson et al. (1993); 634 post-menopausal female volunteers; average age 71 years; white, healthy, community-living, no functional disability. Fairly sedentary. Average BMI = 26.3, 37.7% of sample with BMI > 27.3 (overweight).	Cross-sectional study. Demographic, medical/health, medications, family history, lifestyle, reproductive history. Body weight, height, waist girth, hip girth, BMI, physical activity assessment (Paffenberger), lipids.	(−) Lack of association between lipid profile, activity level, age, BMI, education, and estrogen use. Caution using different physical activity tools (daily tasks of living vs. recreation). Paffenbarger Activity Questionnaire may be inappropriate to use in a sedentary population or low-intensity participation. Recall, self-report, and retrospective data collection raises suspicion, especially in elderly.

(Continued)

Table 2-7
(*Continued*)

Researchers and sample	Measures	Findings
Gardner & Poehlman (1993); 167 volunteers ($n = 111$ equation, $n = 56$ cross validation); 18 to 81 average = 43 to 44 yrs; rest/ex, BP, no obesity/diabetes, no smokers; no CHD, normal ECG.	Cross-sectional study at single point. Body density/% fat, skinfold and circumference, VO_2max, leisure time physical activity.	(+) Leisure time physical activity was a predictor of body density, and predicted better for older women and women with low body density.
Kohrt et al. (1992); Young group = ages 18 to 31 (41 sedentary M, 33 sedentary F, 43 trained M, 16 trained F). Old group = ages 58 to 72 (93 sedentary M, 107 sedentary F, 32 trained M, 12 trained F). Healthy, no chronic disease, none obese, non-smokers. Sedentary had no exercise program; trained were competitive (running, cycling, weight lifting, swimming).	Cross-sectional; body density, skinfold (6 sites), compared age and activity groups. Concerns re: underwater method, RV estimate (Brozek formula used for both young and old).	(+) Old sedentary subjects had more fat than young sedentary subjects; less difference between old trained vs young trained. Difference between young and old, trained and sedentary; little difference for peripheral and lower body skinfold, but at central and upper body sites there was a significant difference. Aging people who exercise accumulate less adipose tissue in upper and central body regions.

(*Continued*)

Table 2-7
(*Continued*)

Researchers and sample	Measures	Findings
Nieman et al. (1990); females 74 years of age or older (average age 82 years); 9 active (age range 67 to 92), 6 inactive (age range 74 to 87).	3-day diet, VO₂max, 3-site skinfold, glucose, blood lipid profile.	(−) Habitual moderate cardiorespiratory (CR) exercise in healthy older women was not associated with improved blood lipid or CR capacity. No differences for age, weight, height, BMI, BP. Inactive had more protein and less fat intake. No differences in glucose and blood lipid profile. Hemoglobin/hematocrit less for inactive, tricep skinfold less in active, no difference in VO₂max. Small sample, weak body composition measures.

increased sodium retention, low dietary intake of calcium, obesity, lack of physical activity, smoking, hyperlipidemia, elevated cholesterol, and atherosclerosis. This section will focus on the effects of physical activity on blood pressure in the elderly.

Blood pressure (especially systolic and mean arterial) and total peripheral resistance increase with age and are higher at the same exercise intensity in the older adult (Julius et al., 1967; Martin et al., 1991). This is primarily the result of a decrease in vascular elasticity and vasodilation capacity. It may also be the result of other related factors such as a decrease in general fitness, a decrease in lean body mass, and various disease-related factors associated with aging that lead to an increased sedentary lifestyle. The age-related increase in blood pressure has been shown to be greater in women than men (Martin et al., 1991; Hossack & Bruce, 1982) and may be related to a decrease in estrogen levels in women (Martin et al., 1991; Luotola, 1983).

One longitudinal study (Kasch et al., 1988) has shown that physical activity may forestall the age-related increase in arterial pressure. Several other shorter-term studies showed aerobic endurance-trained aged athletes to have lower resting and exercise blood pressure at the same submaximal power output in comparison to age-matched untrained elderly subjects or younger subjects (Kasch et al., 1990; Rogers et al., 1990; Martin et al., 1991). Martin et al. (1991) found that endurance-trained older women did not have lower blood pressure during submaximal exercise in comparison to age-matched untrained women. Reaven et al. (1991) reported that lower systolic and diastolic blood pressures were significantly associated with increased activity intensity in the elderly. Lower submaximal exercise blood pressures in the trained male elderly may be the result of an enhanced vasodilatory capacity and/or decreased sympathetic stimulation of vascular tone that occurs with training (Martin et al., 1991).

Some controversy exists as to the effectiveness of aerobic endurance training for correcting hypertension in the aged. Some research has shown a decrease in resting systolic (Singh et al., 1993; Steinhaus et al., 1990), diastolic (Singh et al., 1993; Howze et al., 1989) and mean blood pressure (Webb et al., 1993), and in submaximal exercise blood pressure after training (Martin et al., 1991; Seals et al., 1984). Other research has not shown a significant decline in resting or submaximal blood pressure response with endurance training (Hamdorf et al., 1992, 1993; Adams et al., 1973) despite improved left ventricular function (Ehsani et al., 1991).

The above disparities may be the result of differences or deficiencies in experimental design, training programs (e.g., mode, intensity, duration); blood pressure measurement technique, and whether or not the subjects were normotensive or hypertensive prior to training (Foster et al., 1989; Mayer et al., 1994). Mayer et al. (1994) found both systolic and diastolic blood pressure to be lower after a health program intervention that included an increase in physical activity. There has also been some research that has shown a significant decrease in mean arterial pressure and systemic vascular resistance index with a combined nutrition and exercise program in a sample of obese and hypertensive people that included aged subjects (Weber et al., 1983; Mattar et al., 1990).

Aging has been associated with an increased possibility of postural or orthotic hypotension in the elderly when assuming an upright position (Petrella et al., 1989; Jonsson et al., 1990). The incidence ranges between 11 percent and 30 percent of reported subjects over the age of 61 (Caird et al., 1973; MacLennan et al., 1980). In a review article, Petrella et al. (1989) suggested that the role of physical activity in the management of orthotic hypotension was unclear and required further research.

Table 2-8 illustrates intervention and comparative studies for hypertension outcomes. Table 2-9 shows correlational and epidemiological studies.

Table 2-8
Hypertension Outcomes: Intervention and Comparative Studies

Researchers and sample	Design, treatment, and measures	Findings
Spina et al. (1993); 31 subjects; average age 64 years; 15 male and 16 female, healthy volunteers.	Six men and 10 women in exercise group; 9 men and 6 women served as controls; 2 to 3 months initial flexibility training followed by 9 to 12 months of endurance training consisting of walking, jogging, rowing, cycling; 45 minutes/day, 5 times/ week. Initial intensity 60%–70% of max HR, progressed to 75%–85%. Measured resting systolic and diastolic BP, VO_2max, Q, SV, a-v O_2 difference.	(+) Significant decrease in diastolic blood pressure in women. (−) No change in systolic or diastolic in men and no change in systolic in women. Small sample.
Hamdorf et al. (1992); 80 subjects; average age 64.1 years both groups; volunteers, all women.	Trained group exercised twice a week for 6 months; progressed from 16 to 45 min; used target heart rate zones; 10 dropped out of trained group and 4 dropped out of control group. 90.6% adherence rate for training. Measured heart rate, blood pressure, spirometry variables.	(−) No change in resting systolic or diastolic BP.
Ehsani et al. (1991); 10 subjects; average age 64 years (range of 60 to 70 years).	All subjects performed endurance exercise, 4 days/wk for 1 year; Progressively overloaded from 60% to 80% of VO_2max and some brief bouts at 93% of VO_2max; 3 subjects dropped out for reasons not related to the study. Measured VO_2max, submaximal exercise, left ventricular systolic function, % fat, BP, SV.	(+) Significant increases in VO_2max. Submaximal HR and rate-pressure product were significantly decreased. (−) No change in systolic BP. Improvements in left ventricular systolic performance were noted.

(Continued)

Table 2-8
(Continued)

Researchers and sample	Design, treatment, and measures	Findings
Weber et al. (1983); 70 subjects, 43 men, 27 women; average age 78.7 (range 70 to 88); enrolled in the Pritikin residential program.	26-day Pritikin diet and exercise program; walking 2 times/day for 15–30 min at 70%–85% of age-predicted HRmax, increased to 30–40 min, 2 times/day. Also 20–40 min of aerobic calisthenics 5 times/wk. Measured resting and exercise BP, body weight; blood glucose, cholesterol, triglycerides, walking and treadmill performance.	(+) Significant increase in distance walked and METS (intensity) achieved on treadmill. Significant decrease in blood glucose, cholesterol, body weight, resting BP, & exercise systolic BP (latter improved only for men).

COGNITIVE AND PSYCHOMOTOR OUTCOMES

Summary

The overall level of evidence for positive cognitive and psychomotor outcomes of active living among older adults is **indicative**. However, the level of evidence varies by type of outcome and research design. The majority of correlational studies indicate that physically active people experience a slower decline of cognitive functioning with age than their sedentary counterparts. Exercise intervention studies aimed at improving cognitive functioning in previously sedentary elderly have been inconclusive. There is some indication that exercise can improve cognitive functioning; however, it is unclear what the necessary parameters are that will allow such improvement to occur.

The relationship between an active lifestyle and preservation of cognitive abilities needs to be studied further with a view to establishing the causal direction of this relationship. Longitudinal studies that involve people at a younger age and consider such factors as education, gender, socioeconomic status, and intelligence and other cognitive abilities, are needed in this area.

More uniformity in measures of cognitive functioning, exercise, active living and physical fitness is desirable. For example, different assessments of aerobic capacity yield different results (Era et al., 1986). Since the effect of physical activity on cognitive function is hypothesized to be general rather than specific

Table 2-9
Hypertension Outcomes: Correlational and Epidemiological Studies

Researchers and sample	Measures	Findings
Martin et al. (1991); sedentary and trained (runners) men and women ages 60 to 69, 16 in each group; The older female athlete group consisted of subjects who had just completed an 8-month endurance training program.	Height, weight, % fat, resting and exercise BP, treadmill time, VO_2max, HRmax, RERmax, calf blood flow and conductance.	(+) Trained older men had lower mean BP than sedentary men during submax and max exercise, and lower systolic BP during submax exercise. Max calf blood flow, conductance higher in athletic men, athletic women. (−) No link between exercise and reduced BP for women. Submax and max exercise systolic BP significantly higher in sedentary older women than men. Older trained men and women did not significantly differ in resting BP.
Reaven et al. (1991); 641 Caucasian women; 50 to 89 years; subjects part of Hypertension Detection and Follow-up Program in southern California since 1972. Upper-middle-class. Assessed 1984–1987.	Resting HR, BMI, lifestyle factors and activity questionnaire, BP, medication history, CHD incidence, medical history. Physical activity was classified as none, light, moderate, heavy.	(+) Routine physical activity by older women associated with lower blood pressure, lower resting HR, lower prevalence of hypertension.
Kasch et al. (1990); 18-year study of 15 male exercisers (initial age 44.6), 15 nonexercisers (initial age 51.6). Subjects were healthy volunteers.	Training diary kept by subjects. Resting blood pressure measured.	(+) Resting BP did not change in the exercise group and was significantly higher in the nonexercise group at final testing. The nonexercising group was older.

(Continued)

Table 2-9
(Continued)

Researchers and sample	Measures	Findings
Sedgwick et al. (1988); 290 women; 20 to 65 years; subjects had previously joined a fitness program. After 5 years, divided into active group (vigorous exercise 2 times/wk) or inactive group. 496 initially contacted, of these 364 were contacted after 5 years. 290 (80%) attended the follow-up.	Age, height, weight, BMI, BP, triglycerides, cholesterol. Active group differed significantly from inactive for weight, BMI, diastolic BP (not systolic), triglycerides.	Physical activity and a change in fitness was only weakly related to changes in BP (hypertension). Admitted sample bias in social characteristics and health consciousness.

(Salthouse, 1988), it may be useful to combine a number of (standard) cognitive tests into a composite measure rather than measuring a great number of single tests. Research designs can be improved by attending to such factors as random assignment to conditions, tester's blindness to experimental conditions, sufficient sample sizes to detect smaller effects, use of attention control groups, and direct measures of fitness improvements. More insight into cognitive and movement effects can be attained if reaction time (RT) measures are fractionated into premotor time (PMT), contractile time (CT), and movement time (MT).

Rather than focusing solely on healthy subjects who may show little improvement, future research may also include less healthy elderly, in particular, elderly with cognitive impairments. It would also be useful to investigate the relationship of physical activity not only with laboratory measures of cognitive and motor functioning, but also with measures that have more direct relevance to cognitive and physical functioning in everyday life.

Finally, the finding that individuals who maintain an active lifestyle throughout their lives also appear to preserve a higher level of cognitive functioning implies that it may be better to become active early in life and sustain that lifestyle than to try and make up for the loss later on.

Discussion of the Evidence

Cognitive functioning. The major theoretical notion underlying the research on the relationship between physical activity and cognitive functioning is that exercise contributes to better aerobic capacity which in turn leads to greater cerebral blood flow and enhanced neurotransmitter metabolism (Emery & Blumenthal, 1991; Era et al., 1986; Stones & Kozma, 1989). Increased activation of the central nervous system (CNS), in particular neural activation and stimulation of the reticular activating system, is thought to lead to improved attentional focus (Stelmach, 1994). Level of cognitive functioning has been measured through three types of assessment instruments:

(a) cognitive tests,
(b) simple or choice reaction time measures, and
(c) electrophysiological and neurophysiological measures.

There is considerable consensus in the literature regarding the correlation between higher levels of physical fitness and better cognitive performance. The majority of the studies comparing active elderly to elderly with an inactive lifestyle have found that the physically fit individuals perform significantly better on at least some cognitive tasks than the unfit or inactive. Most studies summarized in Tables 2-10, 2-11, and 2-12 reported a positive relationship between physical fitness and cognitive functioning. This relationship has been found consistently, even though the studies have been varied both in the measures of active living and the measures of cognitive functioning.

However, the correlational nature of this evidence prevents any conclusions regarding causality. Although on theoretical grounds it may seem plausible that a higher level of physical fitness can offset the age-related decline in cognitive functioning, it also may be true that people who function better cognitively are more inclined to engage in physical activity.

Intervention studies have examined whether exercise programs can improve the cognitive functioning of previously sedentary elderly. However, the results of these studies have so far been inconclusive. Of over 30 studies (A.L.C.C.O.A., 1995), 28 found a small to moderate positive effect on cognitive functioning following an exercise program (most noticeably, Dustman et al., 1984); five found no effect at all. Of the latter, the Blumenthal et al. (1991) study has been the most extensive and widely cited.

Many possible explanations have been offered for the inconsistent results of the intervention studies. The effect may be task-dependent, in that the effect may be stronger for more cognitively complex tasks or tasks that require effortful processing than for simpler or more automatized tasks (see Chodzko-Zajko & Moore, 1994, for a discussion of task demands and their effect on cognitive performance). Also, there may be a ceiling effect for cognitive functioning, in that if subjects are functioning at a relatively high cognitive level at the beginning of an exercise program, there is not much room for improvement. Also, there may be a ceiling effect for aerobic fitness, in that cognitive functioning may not improve beyond a certain level of fitness.

There may be a threshold for aerobic fitness improvement, in that cognitive functioning may not improve below a minimum increase in fitness. Related to this latter factor is the duration of the intervention program. It may not be long enough to have an effect on cognitive functioning.

Age may determine whether an intervention can have an effect. If subjects are too young, the decline in cognitive functioning may not be great enough to allow measurable improvement; if subjects are very elderly, the decline may either be too severe to arrest, or physical frailty may prevent significant improvements in aerobic fitness from occurring. Moreover, the effect size may be so small that sample sizes are not sufficient to detect it. Finally, many studies suffer from methodological flaws, such as non-random assignment to experimental and control groups, examining a large number of dependent variables with only a small sample size.

A few studies have looked at the effects of a bout of short-term (rather than chronic) exercise on cognitive functioning, in particular, among the frail elderly and elderly with memory problems (Table 2-12). Some temporary effects have been noted. This type of research may shed light on the value of short and non-strenuous exercise sessions before cognitively demanding situations, but further studies are needed. Another aspect worthy of further investigation is the extent to which improvements in cognitive functioning actually enhance functional behavior in everyday life.

Motor functioning and reaction time. Studies in this area have focused on reaction time tasks consisting of two components: reaction time (RT) and movement time (MT). RT can further be divided into pre-motor time (PMT: the time from the presentation of the stimulus to the arrival of the neural impulse to the motor point) and contractile time (CT: the time from the neural impulse to the initiation of the movement, also called motor time). MT is the time needed to carry out the motor response (i.e., the time of actually moving the limb). RT is generally interpreted as a measure of cognitive functioning, because it represents the speed of information processing. For this reason, RT has been included in the overview of studies on cognitive functioning.

The motor components of RT tasks can only be studied if RT is fractionated so that PMT, CT, and MT are measured separately. Many studies that include RT tasks do not use fractionated RT. The only distinction that is made is between simple RT (SRT) and choice RT (CRT), with the CRT supposedly measuring a greater cognitive component. However, it is hard to say whether exercise has a greater effect on CRT or SRT. The majority of the correlational studies involving

RT measures have found that active elderly outperform their non-active peers on both SRT and CRT measures, but experimental studies have found significant and nonsignificant effects for SRT and CRT in almost equal numbers.

Of the studies that used fractionated RT measures, most correlational studies showed that active elderly had faster total RTs as well as MTs and PMTs. Two studies found that they were not faster on CT. None of the experimental studies that included fractionated measures found significant effects. This may suggest that the influence of exercise may be felt both in the cognitive component of RT tasks and the movement component, but maybe not as much in the contractile component. More studies using fractionated measures are needed, to shed a light on this issue.

Very few tasks other than straight RT tasks have been used to study the effect of exercise on psychomotor skills of the elderly. Some researchers have studied tapping tasks (Era et al., 1986; Stones & Kozma, 1988), and one study employed a clothespin hand/arm coordination task (Puggaard et al., 1994). Stones & Kozma (1988) suggested that overlearned motor activities will not decline with age. Some attention has been paid to the relationship between physical fitness and motor learning (Del Rey, 1982). The results suggest that such a relationship exists; physically fit elderly learn a new motor task faster and better than their less fit counterparts. Further research in this area should focus on the effects of specific fitness atrributes on learning new tasks.

Tables summarizing studies of cognitive and psychomotor functioning appear in the pages that follow. Table 2-10 illustrates experimental (intervention) studies of the effects of physical activity on cognitive functioning; Table 2-11 focuses on correlational studies. Table 2-12 focuses on intervention studies of the effects of physical activity on reaction time.

The following is a glossary of abbreviations used in the tables:

- STM: Short-Term Memory
- SRT: Simple Reaction Time
- CRT: Choice Reaction Time
- DRT: Discriminatory Reaction Time
- PMT: Pre-Motor Time: central processing component; time from onset of stimulus to the appearance of an action potential in the muscle
- CT: Contractile Time (also sometimes referred to as Motor Time): peripheral component; time from the arrival of the action potential to the initiation of the movement
- total RT: total Reaction Time, consisting of PMT and CT
- MT: Movement Time: time needed to actually execute the movement
- HR: Heart Rate

Table 2-10
Cognitive Outcomes: Intervention and Comparative Studies

Researchers and sample	Design, treatment, and measures	Findings
Emery (1994); 64 subjects (29F, 35M); 53 to 82 years; 32 younger-old (19F, 13M), average age = 61.8; 32 old-old (10F, 22M); average age = 73.1; chronic obstructive pulmonary disease (COPD) patients in outpatient rehab. program (convenience sample).	Intervention of 4 hours of respiratory therapy, warm-up floor exercises, 45 min aerobic (walk, bike and arm erg.); upper-body strengthening; 5 times per week for 1 month; 3 dropouts; forced vital capacity (FVC) & forced expired volume (FEV); VO_2max (bicycle); distance covered in 12 min walk; digit symbol (WAIS-R); digit span (WAIS-R); trail making; finger tapping.	(+) Both groups improved significantly on VO_2max; younger-old significantly more than old-old; both groups improved significantly on trail making; younger-old improved significantly more on digit span than old-old; trend towards greater improvement in fingertapping for old-old than younger-old on non-dominant hand.
Hill et al. (1993); 121 subjects (61F, 60M), ages 60 to 73; Average age = 64 years; not exercising; Caucasian; 64% were professionals.	Intervention study with 87 experimental subjects, 34 controls (no exercise). 30 to 50 minutes, 3 to 5 times per week for 9 to 12 months of aerobic exercises and flexibility training. Assessed HRmax; blood pressure (SBP, DBP); VO_2max; short-term memory (STM); working memory; psychomotor speed (cross-off task) and general well-being.	(−) No significant improvements in cognitive function for the exercise group; (+) significant increase in VO_2max in exercise group; modest decrease in DBP; controls significantly decrease on STM.

(Continued)

Table 2-10
(*Continued*)

Researchers and sample	Design, treatment, and measures	Findings
Hawkins et al. (1992). 40 subjects (30F, 10M); ages 63 to 82; healthy volunteers, with self-reported good hearing and normal vision.	Intervention study with 20 exercisers, 20 controls (no exercise); 45 min. aquatics 3 times per week for 10 weeks; 2 dropouts from each group. Measures: time-sharing task; attentional flexibility task.	(+) Significant improvement (decrease) in RT for exercisers, but not for control group. (+) Significant improvement in attentional flexibility for exercises only. (−) No significant effect on single tasks, only on more complex attentional tasks.
Chodzko-Zajko et al. (1992). 49 subjects (31F, 18M); 13 young (18 to 27 years), 23 middle-age (50 to 65 years), 13 old (65 to 88 years). Convenience samples, 2 years college education, no depression.	Comparative study of middle-age and older groups who were re-grouped into 18 low-fit (average age of 66) and 16 high-fit (average age of 60). Measures: frequency-of-occurrence memory, location memory, effortful processing, auditory free recall.	(+) Significant difference in free recall memory; high-fit performed better than low-fit. (−) No differences between fitness groups or other memory measures.
Shay and Roth (1992); 105 males. Three age ranges 18 to 28, 35 to 45, 60 to 73. Volunteers recruited from local community groups, athletic clubs, intro. psych classes, track club members. Healthy.	Comparison of high-fit and low-fit in 3 age groups: 15 young high-fit, 17 young low-fit; 17 middle high-fit, 18 middle low-fit; 19 old high-fit, 19 old low-fit. Level of fitness determined on basis of self-reported activity + VO_2max (estimated on basis of submax bicycle test). Measured WAIS-R vocabulary as a control for intelligence (used as a covariate). Visuo-spatial; attention/concentration; verbal memory; simple sensorimotor tasks.	(+) Significant difference between high and low fitness groups only on the visuo-spatial tasks, in particular: old high-fit performed significantly better than old low-fit. (−) Differences in performance between high-fit and low-fit in the middle group were smaller and non-significant, and even smaller and non-significant in the young group.

(*Continued*)

Table 2-10
(Continued)

Researchers and sample	Design, treatment, and measures	Findings
Blumenthal et al. (1991); 101 subjects (51F, 50M), ages 60 to 83; healthy, free from CHD; sedentary.	Intervention study: All subjects randomly assigned to groups; 33 aerobic (AE), avg. age $= 66.5$; 34 yoga (YO), avg. age $= 67.8$; 34 waiting list (WL), avg. age $= 68.8$. AE: 10 min. warm-up, 30 min. bicycling $+$ 15 mild jogging, 5 min. cool-down. YO: 60 min. yoga. WL: no exercise. AE: 3 times per week; YO: 2 times per week both for 16 weeks after 16 weeks (T2). All subjects participated in an aerobic exercise program for 16 weeks (T3), and a majority for another 6 months (T4); 4 dropouts before; T2 ($n = 97$); 7 dropouts between T2 and T3 ($n = 90$); Measured anxiety, depression, mood; psychiatric symptoms; finger tapping; memory: Randt, digit span (WAIS-R); Benton and selective reminding test; perceptual motor: digit symbol (WAIS-R), trail making, 2 and 7 test.	$(-)$ Correlations between changes in VO_2max and changes in psychological functioning between T1 and T4 were small and not significant. $(+)$ Aerobic exercise was associated with a significant increase in VO_2max, which was maintained and increased among subjects who continued to exercise (up to 18%). All subjects, independent of their exercise pattern, improved their perceptual motor functioning over time (practice effect).

(Continued)

Table 2-10
(*Continued*)

Researchers and sample	Design, treatment, and measures	Findings
Stevenson and Topp (1990); 72 subjects (40F, 32M); healthy volunteers; ages 60 to 81; 77% married, 96% Caucasian, 67% some post-high school education; mostly middle and upper- middle socio-economic levels.	Intervention study: one hour of stretching, calisthenics, stationary bike and walking, 3 times per week for 9 months. 39 participants in moderate intensity program; 33 in low intensity. Measured subjective well-being: life satisfaction; perception of health; sleep patterns; mental status: orientation; attention/concentration; STM, higher cognitive functioning (subtests of WMS); cardiovascular fitness, blood pressure, VO_2max.	(+) Both groups improved significantly on attention/concentration, STM, and higher cognitive function. Both groups improved significantly on quantity of sleep and future-oriented health perceptions. Both groups showed positive changes in fitness. (−) No significant difference between the 2 groups in the degree of improvement.
Dustman et al. (1990); 60 males. Young = age 20 to 31, old = age 50 to 62. Volunteers solicited by newspaper; healthy, nonsmoking.	Comparison study of four groups: 15 young high fit, 15 young low fit; 15 old high fit, 15 old low fit. Fitness level measured by VO_2max (direct); WAIS-vocabulary as a measure of verbal and mental ability; somatosensory and visual sensitivity; EEG and ER. Cognitive tests: Sternberg RT, Stroop color interference, symbol digit, Trails B.	(+) Old high fit significantly higher on WAIS-vocabulary than old low fit and young high fit. (+) Old high fit significantly more years of education than other groups; (+) old low fit significantly longer P300 ERP latency than other groups; (+) cognitive performance better for young than old, and for high fit than for low fit.

(*Continued*)

Table 2-10
(Continued)

Researchers and sample	Design, treatment, and measures	Findings
Dustman et al. (1990); 43 subjects. Ages 55 to 70. Healthy, sedentary community volunteers.	Intervention study with three groups: 13 aerobic, 15 stretching, 15 nonex. control. Aerobic: 1 hr. fast walking, exercise control: 1 hr. stretching and flexibility exercises; 3 times/week for 4 months. Aerobic: 60% to 80%; stretching: lower. Measured VO_2max, cognition: critical flicker fusion (CFF) threshold; simple reaction time (SRT); digit symbol, dots estimation, Stroop color interference.	(+) Aerobic group had VO_2max increase of 27%; stretching group: VO_2max increase of 9%. Aerobic: significant improvement on CCF, SRT, and tests of mental flexibility. (+) Both exercise groups showed significant improvement in combined cognitive test score, greatest for the aerobic group.
Emery and Gatz (1990); 48 subjects (40F, 8M); ages 61 to 86 (avg. age = 72). Ethnically diverse; mostly low and middle-income; 80% no education beyond high school; no participation in regular physical activity prior to study.	Comparative study of three groups: 15 physical exercise; 15 social control; 18 waiting list control. Exercise: 10–15 min of stretching, 20–25 min of aerobic exercise, including rapid walking, 5 min dance and cooling down. Social control: 1 hr of non-physical social activities; 3 times/week for 12 weeks. Nine subjects lost to attrition, 1 from exercise group, 4 from each of control groups; low attendance in social group (social activities already available). Pooled control groups. Measured weight, flexibility, resting HR, resting blood pressure; subjective well-being, locus of control, cognition: digit span, digit symbol (WAIS-R), copying words and numbers.	(−) Very little change on any of the cognitive measures in either group; nothing significant. (+) In exercise group: significant correlation between reductions in diastolic BP with improved writing speed and increased mastery; significant correlation between reduced weight and improved writing speed.

(Continued)

Table 2-10
(Continued)

Researchers and sample	Design, treatment, and measures	Findings
Madden et al. (1989); Sample as described in Blumenthal et al. (1991).	Randomized control study as in Blumenthal et al. (1991). Analyses on 79 subjects. Measured VO$_2$max, letter search (STM processing), word comparison (LTM processing), both tasks involve CRT and SRT.	(−) No significant differences on any of the cognitive variables. (+) Significant increase in VO$_2$max for aerobic exercise group (11% at T2).
Clarkson-Smith and Hartley (1989); 124 (F and M); ages 55 to 91; living independently in community or retirement housing; free from CNS disorders; 99% Caucasian.	Comparative study of 62 most active, 62 least active. Two exercise levels. High: minimum 3100 kcal per week energy expenditure and minimum 1.25 hr./week strenuous exercise. Low: Max. 1900 kcal/wk, max. 10 min/wk exercise. Measured SRT and CRT, vocabulary test; working memory: letter sets, digit span and reading span; reasoning.	(+) Two groups differed significantly on HR and vital capacity. High exercise group performed significantly better in all 3 measures of RT, all 3 tests of reasoning and 2 tests of working memory (letter sets and reading span).
Stones and Kozma (1989); 80 subjects (40F, 40M); avg. age young = 21.2; old = 62.9; volunteers, high educational, occupational status; healthy; absence of uncorrected sensory deficits.	Comparative study: 20 each of young active, young inactive, old active, old inactive. Group assignment based on self-reported activity levels: sedentary < 1.5 kcal/kg/day; active > 1.5 kcal/kg/day. Measured modified digit symbol and symbol digit tasks (coding performance and spatial localization), with low or high task interference (distraction).	(+) Older exercisers performed significantly better than older non-exercisers in symbol digit, but not in the digit symbol task; no effect of task interference; no effect for younger subjects.

(Continued)

Table 2-10
(*Continued*)

Researchers and sample	Design, treatment, and measures	Findings
Stones and Kozma (1988); (Study A) 311 subjects, ages 50 to 86.	Comparative study of four groups: 123 exercise (EX), avg. age = 61.7; 60 waiting list, avg. age = 62.2; 92 controls, avg. age = 62.9; 8 male Master athletes (MA), avg. age = 60.1; 28 elder hostelers (EH), avg. age = 70.7. EX program for persons over 50. Controls (no intention to participate) matched with EX and WL. Measured activity levels, digit symbol (WAIS-R), happiness scale (MUNSH), trait anxiety, psych. hardiness, RT, balance; physiological measures like body mass, BP, vital capacity, trunk forward flexion, hearing loss, presbyopia; standardized test of fitness.	(+) Only EH group significantly different from control group on the digit symbol task; MA and EH significantly different from control group on balance. EX, MA, and EH significantly different from controls on flexibility and an aggregate functional age index (consisting of balance, flexibility, digit symbol, and vital capacity).
Molloy et al. (1988); 45 F (initially 50); ages 73 to 90. Nursing home residents, relatively healthy, able to walk, free from disability or disease.	Comparative study of two groups: 23 exercise (avg. age = 82); 22 controls (avg. age = 83.3). Program aimed at improving balance, coordination, and muscle strength, not aerobic fitness. Progress 10 to 35 min; 3 times/week for 3 months; 2 dropouts from exercise, 3 from control. Measured immediate recall, total recall, recognition, digit symbol (WAIS-R), digit span (WAIS-R), logical memory (WMS), word fluency, mini mental state.	(+) Significant improvement in the word-fluency test. (−) No significant improvement for any of the other tests.

(*Continued*)

Table 2-10

(*Continued*)

Researchers and sample	Design, treatment, and measures	Findings
Dustman et al. (1984); 43 subjects (16F, 27M); ages 55 to 70. Healthy, sedentary.	Intervention study with random assignment to aerobic and strength groups, not to control group. 13 aerobic (avg. age = 60.6), 15 strength and flexibility (avg. age = 62.3), 15 controls (avg. age = 57.4). Aerobic: fast walking and slow jogging. Strength and flexibility; 1 hour per session; 3 times/week for 4 months. Up to 70% to 80% HRR for aerobic group, strength group below that. No dropouts reported. Measured CFF, IQ, digit span, digit symbol, dots estimation, RT, Stroop.	(+) VO_2max improvement significantly greater for aerobic than strength group (27% vs. 9% increase). Significantly greater improvement in aerobic group on CFF, digit symbol, dots estimation, Stroop and SRT. Significant improvement in cognitive performance (composite score) for aerobic and strength groups. (−) No improvement in CRT for either group.

BALANCE OUTCOMES

Summary

The level of evidence for balance outcomes is **acceptable**. The majority of studies indicate that balance can be significantly promoted with formal exercise training in inactive, healthy older volunteers. Some studies suggest that specificity of balance training is needed.

Which forms of physical activity make the most significant contributions to balance proficiency is yet to be determined. Although controlled exercise interventions lead to improvement in a variety of balance measures, the outcomes for falls prevention and reduced injury are less clear when compared to other falls reduction strategies.

Balance promotion in frail and/or ill populations is unclear. The frailty and possible lack of motivation of institutionalized elderly limit duration and intensity of exercise sessions, thereby compromising the findings. Also, balance proficiency as an outcome of informal active living is unknown.

Table 2-11
Cognitive Outcomes: Correlational and Epidemiological Studies

Researchers and sample	Measures	Findings
Christensen and Mackinnon (1993); 116 subjects; 60 young, 56 old, > 70, live independently. High educ: old (univ. grads); young educ., Ph.D. students. Old low educ: retired blue collar workers, young low-educ: blue collar workers.	Self-reported activity levels: Schonfield scale + hourly diaries; Cognitive functioning: 4 intelligence tasks, 6 memory tasks: 3 factors: fluid and crystallized intelligence, and memory.	(+) For older subjects, but not for younger, greater physical activity was associated with higher levels of fluid task performance. (−) No significant relationship was found for crystallized intelligence, nor for memory.
Hultsch et al. (1993); 484 subjects (293F, 191M); 106 younger (55 to 64), 256 middle (65 to 74); 58 older, (75 to 86); avg. age = 69.2. Community-dwelling, relatively healthy, average 13.2 years of education.	Self-reported: health status, active lifestyle (incl. physical activity), passive lifestyle, substance abuse, (4 factors in factor analysis), age, semantic processing time, comprehension time, working memory, vocabulary, verbal fluency, world knowledge, word recall, text recall.	Self-reported health and activity lifestyle both predicted cognitive performance even when effects of education, age, and sex have been removed. (+) Correlation of active lifestyle and verbal processing time, vocabulary, and world knowledge significantly higher in older than in middle and younger groups. (+) Higher education correlated with more active lifestyle.
Borchelt and Steinhagen-Thiessen (1992); 450 subjects; (207F, 43M); age 70 to 103; 212 old (avg. age = 77.4; 238 very old (avg. age = 92). Probability sample from the residential registry in West Berlin living in private households and institutions.	Activities of daily living (ADL), max. walking distance, grip strength, digit letter test (like digit symbol).	(+) Walking distance (.33), letter digit (.04), and sensory impairment (.01) together accounted for nearly 40% of variance in ADL status in stepwise regression; walking distance and cognition shared most of the variance they could account for.

(*Continued*)

Table 2-11
(*Continued*)

Researchers and sample	Measures	Findings
Rogers et al. (1990); 83 subjects (30F, 53M); avg. age = 64.4. 27 working (W); avg. age = 64.4; 28 retired high-active (RH); avg. age = 64.9; 28 retired low-active (RL); avg. age = 64.4. Neurologically normal; not retiring for health reasons; healthy. Prospective study; 7 dropouts over 4 years, 3 in working group, 2 each in retirement groups (initial *N* was 90).	Compared working vs. active and inactive retirees; cognitive capacity screening examination (CCSE); cerebral blood flow (CBF).	(+) CBF values decreased significantly over time for RL, not for W or HL; significantly lower CCSE scores for RL after 4 years than W or HL. No significant changes in activity levels over time between RH and RL.
Clarkson-Smith and Hartley (1990); 300 subjects; Ages 55 to 91 (213F, 87M). Living independently in community or retirement housing; free from CNS disorders; 99% Caucasian.	Age, self-rated health, education. Kcal per week exercise expenditure; kcal per week activity; forced expiratory volume; HR, DBP, SBP. Cognitive: SRT and CRT (2/4 choice) (finger); letter sets (memory); WAIS-R digit span backwards; reading span; analogies; matrices; letter series.	(+) LISREL analysis supported the hypothesis of a positive relationship between exercise and cognition. Effect of exercise on cognitive performance independent of health; age-related deficits in cognition cannot be completely explained by impaired health and decreased physical activity.
Cockburn et al. (1990); 119 subjects (75F, 44M); ages 77 to 94, avg. age = 80.5; 85 subjects recruited by random selection from GP register, 34 from people living at home or attending geriatric day hospital, 2 months.	Frenchay Activities Index (FAI); Barthel Index for ADL; National Adult Reading Test (NART); Rivermead Behavioral Memory test (RBMT); Raven's colored program matrices.	(+) Raven's test significantly associated with FAI items: light housework, gardening, household/car maintenance. RBTM significantly associated with heavy housework, shopping, walking outdoors, hobbies.

Table 2-12

Reaction Time Outcomes: Intervention and Comparative Studies

Researchers and sample	Design, treatment, and measures	Findings
Lord and Castell (1994); 84 subjects (67F, 17M), ages 50 to 75, avg. age = 62.4. Living independently in a community in Australia; not free of diseases like high BP, osteoarthritis, heart disease, diabetes; control group drawn from a different study.	Intervention study. Two groups: 44 exercise, 40 control (all F). Exercise: 1 hr. warm-up, walking, gentle exercise (flex. and strength); subjects encouraged to continue other physical activities 2 times per week for 10 weeks. 4 subjects not retested, analysis on $n = 40$. Measured quadriceps strength, SRT (foot, body sway: on firm surface and on foam with eyes open and closed.	(+) Significant improvement on quadriceps strength, SRT, body sway on firm surface with eyes closed and body sway on form with eyes open and closed.
McMurdo and Rennie (1994); 65 subjects (54F, 11M), ages 67 to 89. Residents of senior homes in Scotland; subjects able to toilet, dress, and walk independently, but no screening for medical conditions.	Intervention study. Random assignment to groups: 36 exercise (avg. age = 83.7), 29 reminiscence (avg. age = 82). Exercise: progress to 45 min seated isometric exercises to music. Controls: 45 min reminiscence therapy twice/week for 6 months; 4 dropouts from exercise group; 6 dropouts from control. Measured quadriceps muscle strength; step test; CRT: recognition MT and total RT; Mini Mental State (MMSE).	(−) No significant improvements in CRT; MMSE declined more for the control group, but did not reach significance. Significantly higher quadriceps strength at post-test for exercise group vs. control.

(Continued)

Table 2-12

(*Continued*)

Researchers and sample	Design, treatment, and measures	Findings
Puggaard et al. (1994); 59 subjects (F42, 17M), ages 60 to 82. Not participating in regular exercise in past 5 years. Free of major physical problems; living at home in Copenhagen, Denmark. Control group slightly younger than other two groups and still working.	Intervention study. Non-random assignment to one of three groups (subjects' own choices): 19 gymnastics, 11 swimming, 15 senior dance, 14 control. Gymnasts: 45 min, walking/jogging, strength, balance, relaxation. Swimmers: 25 min water gymnastics and swimming. Dancers: 45 min; group dancing various intensity. Frequency: 3 times per week for gymnasts and dancers, 2 times per week for swimmers for 5 months. Intensity: 55% to 74% in gymnasts; 59% to 76% in swimmers; 43% to 81% in dancers. 9 dropouts from training groups; 3 dropouts from control group; health or personal reasons. Measured hand/arm coordination: clothespin test; SRT with hand and foot reacting to visual and auditory stimuli; VO_2max.	(+) Improved hand and arm coordination for both active males and females; improved SRT for hand-to-visual and foot-to-auditory stimuli for active females only; no changes for active males or control. (+) Increased max. voluntary contraction of 7% to 28% in muscle groups studied, in activity groups, not in control; a positive correlation between handgrip strength and coordination for females. (−) No significant improvement in VO_2max.
Lupinacci et al. (1993); 56 subjects (28F, 28M); self-reported health status above average; all subjects univ. professors with Ph.Ds; high active: at least 5 years regular aerobic activity (3 times/week).	Comparative study. Four groups: 14 old, high active (avg. age = 58.4); 14 old, low active (avg. age = 58.7); 14 young high active (avg. age = 40.1); 14 young low active (avg. age = 43.4). Measured self-reported activity levels; SRT and CRT (finger); digit symbol (WAIS).	(+) Activity effect, for both age groups, on SRT and CRT: high active performed better. No significant age x activity level interactions. Digit symbol differences greater between high and low active older than younger subjects but not significant.

(*Continued*)

Table 2-12
(*Continued*)

Researchers and sample	Design, treatment, and measures	Findings
Voorrips et al. (1993); 50 females, ages 60 to 80. Healthy volunteers; independently living; medium-sized city in The Netherlands.	Comparative study of three groups: 19 most active, 15 intermediate, 16 least active. Self-reported activity levels: high, medium, low. Measured SRT to light stimulus, manual dexterity, grip strength.	(−) No significant differences in SRT, manual dexterity, or grip strength.
Lord et al. (1993); 42 females, ages 57 to 75; Australia.	Intervention study. Two groups: 21 exercise, 21 control, 1 hr. of gentle aerobic exercise, emphasizing balance and flexibility; 2 times per week for 12 months 60% + VO_2max. Measured quadriceps strength, ankle dorsiflexion strength, proprioception, SRT (finger), body sway.	(+) Exercisers performed significantly better on quad strength, RT, and body sway (on foam with eyes closed).
Hassmen et al. (1992); 32 females; young old ages 55 to 65, old-old 66 to 75. Healthy volunteers.	Intervention study. Exercise and control groups for each age group (8/group). Exercise: 20 minutes walking. 3 times per week for 3 months according to RPE scale (ratings of perceived exertion). Controls: mental arithmetic. 2 dropouts due to illness, analyses on $n = 30$. Measured face recognition, SRT and CRT (finger), estimated VO_2max, SBP and DBP, digit span (STM), HR.	(+) All groups had faster CRTs at post-test, exercise groups had improved significantly more; significant improvement in digit span for exercise groups. (−) No significant improvement in estimated VO_2max; significant improvement in HR; no significant effects for SRT, or on the face recognition task.

(*Continued*)

Table 2-12
(*Continued*)

Researchers and sample	Design, treatment, and measures	Findings
Rikli and Edwards (1991); 48 F, ages 57 to 85. Self-reported health, free of physical ailments; no regular exercise involvement in last 15 years; volunteers.	Non-random assignment to groups: 31 exercise (ages 57 to 85), 17 control (ages 59 to 81). Exercise: 5–10 min warm-up, 20–25 min aerobics, 20–25 min calisthenics, 5–10 min cool down. Controls: hobby class (no exercise) 3 times per week for 3 years, 60% to 70% intensity. 80% compliance, 10 dropouts from exercise group, 4 dropouts from control; analyses on $n = 21$ and 13. Measures: 2 min step test; SRT and CRT; static balance; flexibility; grip strength.	(+) Significant improvements on CRT, balance, flexibility, and grip strength, not on SRT after 1 year. (−) No significant changes from year 1 to year 3. Controls experienced declines, except on grip strength.
Whitehurst (1991); 14 F, ages 61 to 73, avg. age = 65.8. Healthy, sedentary, rural community, own household, active in community.	Intervention study. Randomly assigned to exercise or control groups ($n = 7$ in each). Exercise: aerobic, bicycle erg. starting 8–10 min up to 35–40 min at end. 3 times per week for 8 weeks at 70% to 80% of individual VO_2max. Controls: no exercise. Measures: simple reaction time (SRT), choice reaction time (CRT), VO_2max.	(−) No significant differences between exercisers and control in SRT or CRT; (+) Significant increase in VO_2max for exercisers at post, not for control.

(*Continued*)

Table 2-12
(*Continued*)

Researchers and sample	Design, treatment, and measures	Findings
Panton et al. (1990); 49 subjects (26F, 23M), ages 70 to 79; retired professionals recruited from university community; sedentary non-smokers; healthy.	Intervention study. Three groups: 17 walk/jog, 20 strength training, 12 controls. Aerobic: progressive, 20 min to 45 min walking/jogging. Strength: 30 min resistance Nautilus exercise machines. Control: no exercise. Program 3 times/week for 26 weeks. Intensity: aerobic, start at 50% up to 75% to 85% of HRRmax; strength, 8–12 reps, progressively heavier. 57 subjects started program, i.e., 8 dropouts. Measured VO_2max, strength, premotor movement time (PMT), total RT (SRT), MT.	(+) Significant increase in VO_2max in walk/jog group, not in control or strength groups; low but significant correlation between changes in VO_2max and changes in total RT (SRT). (−) No significant differences between groups on PMT, CT, total RT (SRT), or MT.
Roberts (1990); 61 subjects (52F, 9M), ages 65 to 87, avg. age = 71.8; recruited from 7 senior citizen centers; healthy, sedentary.	Intervention study. Groups: 31 experimental, 30 control. Exp: walking 30 minutes, control: no exercise. Walking 3 times/week for 6 weeks at 60% to 70% of age-adjusted max. heart rate (220-age). 5 subjects lost from control group. 4 lost from exp. Measured SRT and CRT + movement times (MT).	(+) CRT significantly shorter for exp. subjects who walked more miles per week. (−) No significant differences between exp. and control in SRT, CRT, or MT; CRT and SRT significantly slower for subjects with higher index of past aerobic activity.

(*Continued*)

Table 2-12
(*Continued*)

Researchers and sample	Design, treatment, and measures	Findings
Bashore (1989); 140 males, ages 60 to 84 (older); 20 to 35 (younger). Active older: exercised at least the last 10 years; active younger at least 2 years.	Comparative study. Six groups: 60 older (non-exercisers, reaction-time exercisers, involved in racket sports and handball; aerobic exercisers, involved in bicycling and running) 50 younger (also comprised of reaction-time, aerobic, and non-exercisers). Measures: fitness level based on VO$_2$max: hi fit > 35 ml/min/kg; low fit < 25 ml/min/kg, CRT, P300 ERP latency.	(+) The shortest RT of the older low fit comparable to the longest RT of the older hi fit subjects; slowest RT of the older low fit slowest of all groups; hi fit older had shorter P300 latencies than low fit older.
Clarkson-Smith and Hartley (1989); 124 subjects (F + M), ages 55 to 91; living independently in community or retirement housing; free from CNS disorders; 99% Caucasian.	Comparative study. Two groups: 62 most active, 62 least active. High active: min of 3100 kcal per week energy expenditure and minimum of 1.25 hrs./week strenuous exercise. Low active: max. of 1900 kcal/week and max. of 10 min/week exercise. Measured SRT and CRT; vocabulary test; working memory: letter sets, digit span and reading span; reasoning.	(+) High exercise group performed significantly better in all 3 measures of RT, all 3 tests of reasoning, and 2 tests of working memory (letter sets and reading span); two groups differed significantly on HR and vital capacity.

(*Continued*)

Table 2-12
(*Continued*)

Researchers and sample	Design, treatment, and measures	Findings
Bashore et al. (1988); 60 males; ages 60 to 84 (old), 20 to 35 (young); medical screening; active older: subjects had been active in aerobic activities for many years.	Comparative study. Four groups (matched on IQ): 15 old active, 15 old inactive, 15 young active; 15 young inactive. Measured level of fitness; CRT; P300 ERP latency.	(+) Old active significantly faster RT and significantly shorter P300 latencies than old inactive; (no difference between YA and YI on these measures). Old inactive with the highest IQ showed the largest loss in processing speed relative to old active.
Baylor and Spirduso (1988); 16 females; ages 48 to 63. Recruited from previous study.	Comparative study. Experimental: 8 runners (avg. age = 53.4), averaging 30 min. per day, 5 times per week. Controls: 8 women working in community (avg. age = 53.9). Measured SRT with MT, CT & PMT; discriminatory RT (DRT) with MT, CT & PMT both in foot RT tasks; EMG of involved muscles.	(+) Exercisers were significantly faster and less variable on central processing: SRT, DRT, PMT, and peripheral RT: CT and MT. Non-exercisers were especially slower in DRT. Exercise SRT faster than ex. DRT and than non-exercise SRT.
Stones and Kozma (1988); (Study B) 80 subjects (40F, 40M).	Comparative study of four groups: 20 young active phys. ed. students (avg. age = 20.4); 20 young inactive, exercise < 30 min./wk (avg. age = 23.2); 20 old active, exercise at least 45 min. 2 times/wk (avg. age = 61.3); 20 old inactive, exercise < 30 min./wk. Measured hand-tapping, foot-tapping, both tasks up and down tapping, both tasks in decoupled (either limb) or coupled (alternating limbs) condition.	(+) Active groups were significantly faster on decoupled movement, but not on coupled movement. Younger groups were significantly faster on hand-tapping but not on foot-tapping tasks (overlearning effect). No interactions significant beyond first-order level.

(*Continued*)

Table 2-12
(*Continued*)

Researchers and sample	Design, treatment, and measures	Findings
Normand et al. (1987); 24 subjects (18F, 6M), avg. age = 65.7; relatively healthy subjects living at home in Eastern Ontario; socially active. Program initiated and run by seniors' club, not specifically for experiment.	Intervention study. Two groups: 12 exercise 12 control (matched by age and sex). Exercise: 1 hour + encouraged to exercise at home, once per week for 10 weeks. Measured fine motor performance on a discrete pursuit motor task: correct RT, non-overshoot MT, overshoot MT, total RT, error score, overshoot score.	(−) No significant differences between the groups on any of the fine motor measures; not possible to say whether there were any significant changes in aerobic fitness. Note small sample size.

Standardized measures of balance are in development. Balance tests range from very crude one-foot stance with eyes open or closed to sophisticated postural-sway force-platforms. Both types of assessments are sensitive enough to obtain statistical results although the one leg stand was not discriminating enough in one healthy population (Iverson et al., 1990). Standardization of balance assessment would assist research greatly in developing normative data.

Current research is often lacking adequate sample sizes to reach statistical significance and many are lacking generalizability (non-random selection). However, there are some well-designed studies with randomized control groups. Studies of longer duration (more than 6 to 12 weeks) are recommended to assess the ability of older people to adhere to an exercise regimen and also to see how balance improvements may be compromised by age declines. As well, balance *maintenance*, rather than significant improvement, may be a more important health outcome of physical activity involvement. A life course perspective is needed to understand the effects of active living on balance over the life span. If balance can be improved, can it be restored to 100 percent?

Discussion of the Evidence

The evidence is generally in favor of exercise interventions leading to improved balance. Twenty-six exercise intervention studies to promote balance are summarized in Table 2-13. Only four studies found no balance improvement after

Table 2-13
Balance Outcomes: Intervention and Comparative Studies

Researchers and sample	Design, treatment, and measures	Findings
Binder et al. (1994); 15 subjects; ages 66 to 97. Community-dwelling adults with at least one risk factor for falls.	8-week intervention study, no control. 1 hour group exercise class, 3 times/week; Self-monitored at HR < 115; self-paced rest periods. One-year follow-up; 15 of 37 adults completed the exercise program (the rest were refusals, disinterest, medical exclusions). Measured Static Balance (Progressive Romberg test).	(+) Balance improved; Number of Romberg positions performed increased from 3.3 to 4.4 ($p < .001$) with $n = 14$. The active subjects maintained their balance scores at the 1 year post-test.
Clemons and Foret (1994); $N = 20$; 4 M, 16 F, ages 57 to 76 years. Medically screened convenience sample.	8-week intervention study with no control group. Stairmaster exercise for 30 minutes, 3 times/week; 55% to 60% of heart rate reserve. Measured static balance, best of 5 trials on one-legged stork stand, each leg and eyes open and closed (4 measures).	(−) Eight weeks of moderate Stairmaster exercise may enhance PWC in elderly subjects but is not likely to affect static balance.
Hu and Woollacott (1994); Study I; 24 subjects, avg. age = 75.6 years, 65 to 90. Independent community volunteers.	10 day intervention study. Randomized control design, exp. = 12; control = 12. Balance tasks: multisensory (moving) platform balance, soft/firm floor surface, eyes open-closed, head neutral/extended, trained for 1 hour/day for 10 days. Assessment up to 4 weeks after study; 2 exercisers and 2 controls had no pre-test due to a change in test protocol. Measures: one leg balance eyes open and closed; platform sensory test (frequency of "falls" or loss or platform balance; Tandem walking; detraining at day 1, week 1, week 4.	(+) The training group improved under all conditions, with significant balance gains on the foam surface, head back, or eyes closed conditions. Significant differences between exercise and control still existed one month later.

(Continued)

Table 2-13

(*Continued*)

Researchers and sample	Design, treatment, and measures	Findings
Hu and Woollacott (1994); Study 2; sample as above.	10 day intervention study. Experimental and control group, balance tasks as above. Measured compensatory postural responses to horizontal platform perturbations.	(+) Stability training led to significant improvements in balance management. The neck flexor muscle was activated significantly earlier in the training group. Training on a moving platform caused muscle activation and kinematic response latencies to be shortened to a greater degree than in controls.
MacRae et al. (1994); 80 F, 60 years and over. Non-random, recruited from seniors' centers in Los Angeles.	12-month intervention study. Experimental group = 42; controls = 38 (non-random). One-hour sessions, education or exercise program of stand-up, step-up activity; Exercise: 3 days/week; control: 1 hour/week. 26% dropout, 2 deaths. Measured eyes-open static balance = 13 → 21 sec.	(−) Non-significant differences; control group lost balance over time while exercise group maintained balance scores.
Mulrow et al. (1994); 194 older adults. Nursing home residents dependent in at least 2 ADLs.	4-month intervention study. Random assignment to friendly visits (FV) or physical therapy (PT); PT included range of motion, strength, balance, transfer, and mobility exercises. One-on-one therapy exercise or visits 3 times per week. Attendance: PT = 89%; FV = 92%; 5% PT and 9% FV drop-out rate. Measured falls; physical disability; ROM, strength, balance, mobility.	(−) No significant difference in balance, ROM, or strength. (+ n.s.) PT group had 79 falls vs. 60 falls in FV group. The standardized PT program provided only modest mobility benefits for very frail long-stay nursing home residents.

(*Continued*)

Table 2-13
(*Continued*)

Researchers and sample	Design, treatment, and measures	Findings
Puggaard et al. (1994); 59 older adults; avg. age 67 years (range 60 to 82). Sedentary, healthy volunteers.	5-month intervention study. Subjects self-selected into exercise of their choice; 25 to 45 min sessions, gymnastics, swimming, dance; 2 sessions/ week. Attendance ranged from 48% to 98%. Measured eyes-closed static balance, best of 3 tries, Right leg = 3.6 → 4.5 sec.; Left leg = 3.7 → 5.2 sec.	(+) The female activity group improved balance with most of the women being in the gymnastics group. (−) The men did not improve balance, but only 4 men were in the gymnastics program.
Duncan et al. (1993); 39 males. Low, intermediate, or high physical per- formance. 69 years or older (avg. age = 75). Men without significant disease from an ongoing study at Durham, North Carolina, Veterans Affairs Hospital (Convenience sample).	Comparative study. Measured physiological components of postural control; 3 levels of function based on stairs and walking ability walking distance in 6 minutes; functional reach; walk time (10 feet).	(−) Physiological components of postural control rarely differed among the three groups. The results of this study demonstrate that decline in functional mobility in elders without severe pathology may be better explained by the accumulation of deficits.
Judge et al. (1993b); 108 male and female older adults. Avg. age = 74 years. Subjects free of neurological disease.	13-week intervention study. Resistance (R), balance (B), combined training, and control groups. 3 times/week. Measured loss of balance (LOB), center of force displacement during sway-referenced balance testing.	(+) Both R and B improved LOB; B only training group to improve all balance/ sway measures suggesting that B improved strategies of ankle movements (torque) to control body movement. R impro- ved the effectiveness of but did not alter balance strategies.

(*Continued*)

Table 2-13

(*Continued*)

Researchers and sample	Design, treatment and measures	Findings
Judge et al. (1993a); 21 women; avg. age 68 years (range 62 to 75). Mail recruitment of women registered with Hartford Insurance Co. (114 of 1300 responded); 46 excluded for medical reasons; 38 completed screening.	6-month intervention study with randomized control; 12 exercise 9 posture. Exercise: Leg resistance training; 20 min walking, posture, and flexibility. Posture: only posture and flex. 3 times/week; 70% MaxHR four dropouts. All subjects attended 50% of the classes. Measured postural sway using force platform; average 3 trials of double stance eyes open (EO) and eyes closed (EC), single stance upright, and single stance with forward lean.	(+) Significant improvement (18%) for exercisers in combined single stance scores (Non-significant 5% increase in posture group). Sample size was too small to detect significance between the two groups.
Lord et al. (1993); 42 females. Ages 57 to 75. Convenience sample drawn from a larger study on falls.	One-year-intervention study. 21 active women age-matched with 21 inactive controls (non-random assignment). One hour of gentle aerobic exercise emphasizing balance and flexibility; 2 times/week. Goal was 60% of maximum heart rate. Drop-out not reported; adherence to exercise = 80%. Measured proprioception (leg position matching); body sway (firm and foam surfaces, eyes open and closed); Body Mass Index.	(+) Exercisers had better balance performance on all sway scores but only eyes closed on foam were significant due to small sample sizes. (−) No difference in test of proprioception.
McMurdo and Rennie (1993); 49 older adults, avg. age 87 years (range 64 to 91). Dundee, Scotland, random selection from four seniors' residences.	7-month intervention study. Exercise = 15; control (reminiscence) = 26. 45 minutes long, 2 sessions/ week. 41 completed, 5 died, 3 dropouts; 91% attendance at exercise sessions. Measured postural sway using a Wright's ataxiameter, feet one pace apart, eyes open and eyes closed.	(+) Postural sway was improved in both groups, exercise group improved more but this was not significant due to small sample size.

(*Continued*)

Table 2-13
(*Continued*)

Researchers and sample	Design, treatment and measures	Findings
Topp et al. (1993); 63 community-dwelling adults ages 65 and over.	12-week intervention study. Driver education class (18 women, 14 men; avg. age 72.8) or 60-minute strength training (21 women, 10 men, avg. age 69.2). 3 times per week. 94% adherence in control group; 81% completed the exercise; Measured eyes-open Static Balance (EOSB); eyes-closed Static Balance (ECSB), Dynamic Balance (walking backward on a line).	(+) A significant improvement in EOSB for both groups of about 8.5 seconds (test effect); a significant improvement in ECSB for control group only (interaction effect); (−) Dynamic Balance was non-significant.
Voorrips et al. (1993); 50 women, 71.5 years. 100 subjects recruited from various locations and door-to-door, The Netherlands.	Single point in time (comparative study); 3 activity levels (groups) based on self-assessed activity; 19 active women; 13 intermediate; 16 inactive. Measured balance board test up to 30 seconds maximum. Best of 3 trials.	(+ n.s.) More active women had better balance. Significance was not reached due to small sample sizes.
Weiner et al. (1993); 41 men; avg. age 67.3 years (range 40 to 105). Inpatient male veterans.	Intervention study. Groups: 28 therapy group; 13 controls (non-random). Measured functional reach every 4 weeks.	(+) Functional reach was sensitive to therapy and considered an appropriate instrument in clinical settings.

(*Continued*)

Table 2-13
(Continued)

Researchers and sample	Design, treatment, and measures	Findings
Keim et al. (1992); 107 patients; 44 M, 63 F; avg. age 57.5 years (range 21 to 87). Balance-disturbed patients at the Hearing & Balance Center in Oklahoma City.	Variable intervention: Only 54% opted to participate in balance rehab program. Duration was self-paced in a self-directed program with occasional supervision. Cawthorne-Cooksey walking and standing exercises; Zee exercises; twice/day every day for as many weeks as needed to obtain improvement (7–19 weeks; avg. 16 weeks). Etiological diagnosis assisted by computerized dynamic posturography; patient self-reported improvement.	(+) 89% of the participants improved balance.
Sauvage et al. (1992); 13 males. Avg. age 73.4 years. Deconditioned male nursing home residents.	12-week intervention study. Randomized control: exercise = 8; controls = 6; exercise: 30–60 min of aerobic cycling and resistance training, 3 times/week (36 sessions) at 70% MHR; 95% compliance rate; 2 exercisers withdrew due to illness. Measures: Tinetti Mobility Scales (dynamic and static balance); postural excursion score.	(+) The Tinetti Balance items were significantly improved in the exercisers, but no improvement in controls. (+ n.s.) Postural sway also improved only in exercisers but did not reach significance (small sample).
Brown and Holloszy (1991); 74 older adults. Volunteers from St. Louis who were non-smokers, in good health, and free of orthopedic problems.	3-month intervention study 62 exercisers; 30 F, 32 M; 13 control, 6 F, 7 M, 64.6 years (self-selected to groups). Ages 60 to 71. One hour of general exercises 5 days/week (independently paced exercise, no exercise leader). Measured one leg stand, eyes open and eyes closed for up to 60 seconds; two trials of each for the best score.	(+) Significant increases in balance were induced by a low-intensity exercise program. The improvements in balance were accompanied by significant improvements in strength and range of motion.

(Continued)

Table 2-13
(*Continued*)

Researchers and sample	Design, treatment, and measures	Findings
Jirovec (1991); 15 older adults; 14 F, 1 M, 70 to 97 (avg. age = 85.7 years). Cognitively and functionally impaired nursing home residents.	4-week intervention study with no control group. 30 minutes of supervised and assisted walking, 5 days per week. Measures: ability to stand on two feet unassisted, walking distance, speed of walking; ability to rise from a chair unassisted.	(+ n.s.) Unassisted balance time on two legs improved from 24 to 26 seconds, but n.s. possibly due to short intervention period of 4 weeks, cognitive impairments, or small sample size of 15.
Johansson and Jarnlo (1991); 34 females. Avg. age = 70. Healthy, independent-living women, volunteers.	5-week intervention study. Random assignment to groups; 18 to exercise; 16 to controls. Exercise: 60 min of musical walking and arm movements and dance steps, 2 times per week. One dropout due to a fall prior to post-test. Measures: Nine tests of balance to a max. of 30 seconds (one-leg stand with variations); beam walk; maximal walking speed of 30 meters; best of three trials.	(+) No pretraining differences; post-training revealed significant differences for 6 of 9 balance tests; all exercisers made improvements with the best improvements seen in the women starting with the poorest balance scores.
Rikli and Edwards (1991); 48 females; avg. age = 70.2 years (range 57 to 85). Female volunteers who were first-time enrollees in exercise classes taught at a local retirement complex.	3-year intervention study. Two groups: 31 exercisers; 17 controls. One-hour general fitness class following ACSM guidelines, at 60% to 70% MHR, 3 times/week. 10 exercisers and 4 controls were lost due to illness or injury, family problems, death, moving, and loss of interest. Measured one-leg stand eyes open on the preferred foot, best of 3 trials.	(+) Balance was maintained, not improved, in the exercisers whereas the control subjects declined significantly.

(*Continued*)

Table 2-13
(*Continued*)

Researchers and sample	Design, treatment, and measures	Findings
Hopkins et al. (1990); 53 females; avg. age 65 years (range 57 to 77). Sedentary, volunteer, community-dwelling women who expressed interest in low-impact aerobic dance.	12-week intervention study. Randomized to exercise and control groups. Exercise: 50-minute exercise session of walking, stretching, and movement to music 3 times/week. HR = 100–120 bpm. Five exercisers and 7 controls dropped out for personal reasons, but were not significantly different on functional fitness measures at pre-test. Measured one-foot stand to a max. of 30 sec.; average of 3 trials on preferred foot.	(+) A 12% increase in balance time occurred in the exercise group; 0% increase occurred in the control group; muscle strength improved 62% along with significant improvement in hip flexibility. Control group showed decline on most fitness measures. Low-impact aerobic dance is a suitable modality for conditioning elderly women.
Iverson et al. (1990); 54 males; avg. age = 71.2 years (range 60 to 90). Non-institutionalized, recruited from Birmingham, Alabama, seniors' centers and churches; some medical exclusions.	Comparative study among three activity groups. Subjects sorted into 3 groups by reported activity level: mildy active, moderately active, and very active. Measured one-legged stand; Romberg test of balance (heel-toe stance with dominant leg behind); max. of 60 seconds; best score of 3 trials; Torque strength of hip flexion, extension, and abduction.	(+) Significant difference among activity levels on balance, strength measures. One-leg stand was significant related to hip strength. Both balance and strength were predicted by self-reported activity level. The Romberg Balance Test was not discriminating enough for healthy older men (87% completed the 60 sec. heel-toe stand).

(*Continued*)

Table 2-13
(*Continued*)

Researchers and sample	Design, treatment and measures	Findings
Crilly et al. (1989); 50 women (avg. age = 85; range 72 to 92). Residents of sheltered apartments, rest homes, or nursing homes, well enough and mobile enough to attend classes. 117 of 169 residents were eligible, 64 gave consent; 14 last-minute refusals.	3-month intervention study. 15 to 35 minutes of two-leg balances, coordination, flexibility, stand-up strength, ankle strength and relaxation exercise; 3 times/week. Measured postural sway using steel force platform.	(−) There was no significant difference between exercisers and controls on ANY measures and trends were inconsistent. Researchers admitted that their program was undemanding and intended not to improve fitness, but, instead, functional, balance. Researchers believed subjects were not motivated; they "were set in their ways."
Lichenstein et al. (1989); 50 females from two high-rise apartments; women over 65 who were single and living alone. Exercisers were better educated and had better vision.	16-week intervention study. Random selection of apartments; non-random assignment of individuals. Two groups: 26 exercisers (avg. age = 77.5), 24 controls (avg. age = 75.9). 60-minute sessions of balance and stretching exercises. Exercise: two sessions per day, 4 days/week. Response rate was 51% in the control apartments and 59% in the exercise apartments. Measured eyes closed one-foot stand, eyes open one-leg stand, sway measures.	(+) After 4 months, exercisers had less sway scores than controls for the eyes open one-leg stand, but not for eyes closed stand. There was a lack of statistical power to detect between-group differences and inadequate compliance with the exercise program.

(*Continued*)

Table 2-13
(*Continued*)

Researchers and sample	Design, treatment, and measures	Findings
Roberts (1989); 61 seniors from seven seniors' centers (avg. age= 71.8).	6-week intervention study. Self-selected into two groups: exercise: 5 males, 26 females; controls: 4 males, 26 females. Exercise: 30 min of level walking, 3 times/week, at 60% to 70% MaxHR. Five controls and 5 exercisers were drop-outs, various reasons. Measures: Balance Scale (Roberts & Mueller, 1987) which uses eight stances, 4 with eyes open and four with eyes closed. Balance Perception Questionnaire (Roberts, 1989).	(+) Participation in a 6-week program of walking at 60% to 70% of MHR significantly improved balance. (−) The groups did not, however, have any differences in perceptions about balance ability before or after the 6 weeks.

exercise intervention. Specifically, standing balance is not always better in exercisers compared with nonexercisers (Clemons & Foret, 1994; Crilly et al., 1989; Lichenstein et al., 1989; Lord et al., 1993). In the Clemon and Foret study (1994), eight weeks of Stairmaster exercise may not have had adequate variety and specificity for balance promotion. In the Crilly study the duration of the intervention (15 minutes) possibly was inadequate; in the Lichenstein study, there were problems with compliance with the intervention. In the Lord study, the improvements were notable, but sample sizes were too small to obtain statistical significance.

Contemporary researchers are struggling with assessment issues. A number of balance tests have been developed, but there is no standardized or universally accepted measure. Some research has compared balance assessments, and there are promising signs that simple field tests such as "functional reach" (Duncan et al., 1990) may have utility. Sophisticated force platforms measuring postural sway are considered to be "the gold standard" of balance measurement, but this kind of technical equipment is not suited to field research.

The scientific community has considerable interest in falls reduction and identifying risk factors for falls. However, there is a lack of research into relationships among active living, balance performance, falls outcomes, and associated health care costs. Moreover, falls reduction strategies have often focused on environmental hazards as opposed to the intrinsic capabilities of older people. There has been less interest in the relationship of balance maintenance or promotion and their relationship to falls or injury reduction. Scientific assessment of the lifestyle factors which are the best determinants of maintaining and improving balance is lacking.

Balance is the primary variable of interest in few studies; researchers tend to add it to their physiological profile as an "interest" item. Thus we still know little about the relationship of balance promotion and falls reduction. A few studies have examined the relationship between balance proficiency and falls outcomes (Studenski et al., 1991; Topper et al., 1993). This relationship is positive and significant, with fallers predicted by greater postural sway, especially with eyes closed (Lord et al., 1991a, b).

The best sensorimotor predictors of sway on a compliant surface (rubber or foam) may be visual acuity, muscle strength, and reaction time. Exercise improves muscle strength and reaction time, and thus may contribute to a reduction of sway when peripheral sensation and ankle support are challenged. Thus a physically active lifestyle may make an important contribution to stability, particularly when subjects are in environmental situations which are unusual challenges for stability.

Balance as an outcome of active living needs to be a more important focus of intervention research. Sport and exercise programs which are already available in communities need to be assessed for their unique contributions to balance. In addition, the outcomes for balance of late-starting versus lifelong active lifestyles are needed. Large, representative, prospective studies comparing simple approaches to maintaining and improving balance need to be funded. To determine conclusively the role exercise may play in maintaining or improving sensorimotor function in older adults requires randomized controlled studies with large samples of subjects (Lord et al., 1993).

Gender differences have been demonstrated, but the explanation for these differences is not clear. Are women demonstrating poorer balance because of differences in reaction time, strength, and/or range of motion? If so, are these differences attributable to differences in active living patterns of older men and women over their life course or to the fact that women live substantially longer than men?

FALLS OUTCOMES

Summary

The level of evidence for falls outcomes is **indicative** of the fact that less active older adults are more likely to fall. Falls and related injuries as outcomes of active living have not been extensively researched. Several studies show that active elderly are at less risk of falling, though some work suggests that being an active older adult increases risk for falls. Other work suggests that when active older people do fall, their risk of experiencing serious injury may be higher. The majority of experts in the field believe that relationship is causal based on the existing body of evidence, but there are few randomized studies and some potential alternative explanations for findings. Research that would clarify the types of activity that put active older adults at risk of falling is also needed, as is research on the unique contribution of various exercise programs in moderating risk.

Discussion of the Evidence

Falls and related injuries as outcomes of active living have received minimal attention from researchers. Dozens of studies have been published on the etiology of falls in terms of environmental factors, but few have concurrently assessed intrinsic factors. Although a number of studies provide evidence that active individuals fall less, randomized control studies are lacking. Samples are frequently obtained from frail populations who are known to be frequent fallers and thus generalizability to less frail populations is not possible.

A fall is defined as "an event in which the patient came to rest on the floor from a lying, standing, or sitting position" (Kippenbrock & Soja, 1993). Age-related declines in strength, range of motion, reaction time, and proprioception are physiological factors contributing to falls. However, sedentary behavior such as bed rest related to a temporary illness is thought to be a major factor leading elderly adults to fall (Gorbien, Bishop, Beers et al., 1992). Sedentary living leads to outcomes which are risk factors for postural instability: muscle weakness in the legs, slower reaction time, and reduced sensation of position (Lord et al., 1991).

Other factors increasing risk for falls are being older, female, single and/or alone, using medications, having vision impairments, having abnormal blood pressure, living in unsafe environments, and having physical mobility problems. A combination of health difficulties seems to magnify stability problems (Teasdale et al., 1991), yet few studies have controlled for health status.

Although exercise and increased physical activity are occasionally mentioned as likely routes for falls prevention (Sattin, 1992), few intervention studies have been conducted to examine falls reduction as a prospective outcome—an outcome in which the economic and health impact would be considerable. However, some have questioned the cost of rehabilitating frail populations with the goal of increasing balance and reducing falls.

Little is known about the comparative frequency and severity of falls among the elderly during sport and exercise versus settings in which adults are merely ambulating to get from place to place. This information is needed since the prevalent view among public health professionals is that older people would not fall if they did not walk and move about. The fact that the majority of reported falls occur outdoors lends support to the notion that older people are at increased risk if leaving the house (Cwikel, 1992). This finding needs explanation.

For advocates of more active lifestyles, such beliefs by the elderly and professionals who care for them pose a major challenge and exacerbate what is possibly the root of the problem (Gurwitz et al., 1994; Malmivaara et al., 1993; Myers et al., 1991). Factors related to physical inactivity, such as lack of protective muscle tissue, insufficient bone density, and poorly maintained neuromuscular mechanisms add to the seriousness of the injury accompanying a fall.

Lower body muscle strength appears to be important, but more information is needed on the muscle groups most critical to preventing falls. Power in hip flexion may be important to save one's balance in forward tripping and stumbling. Information is lacking about the kinds of mobility (active, passive) and about which joints are most needed to prevent damaging falls. For example, orientation input from the ankle appears to have greater importance for preventing falls compared with having a visual reference (Anacker & Di Fabio, 1992). Also, it appears that proprioception, or awareness of position, can be trained (Meeuwsen et al., 1993).

A few studies have examined the relationship between balance proficiency and falls outcomes (Studenski et al., 1991; Topper et al., 1993). This relationship is positive and significant, with fallers predicted by greater postural sway, especially with eyes closed (Lord et al., 1991a, b). Maki and colleagues warn that a fear of falling is a potentially confounding influence linking measures of postural control and fall outcomes (Maki et al., 1991). Other research has found stronger gait such as faster walking speed and longer stride to be associated with non-fallers (Wolfson et al., 1990).

Research is needed to inform physical therapists, health educators, and fitness leaders about the effectiveness of programs to train older people how to fall with less impact (increased surface area technique), and the effectiveness of differing exercise programs on falling risk and fall outcomes. For example, does aquafit exercise put people at a disadvantage for movement on land because in water they can move slowly and still keep their balance? Tables 2-14 and 2-15 illustrate intervention/comparative and correlational/epidemiological studies, respectively.

INJURY OUTCOMES

Summary

The level of evidence for injury outcomes of active living among older adults is **suggestive**, especially for high-intensity activities. For example, Master's athletes

Table 2-14

Falls Outcomes: Intervention and Comparative Studies

Researchers and sample	Design, treatment, and measures	Findings
MacRae et al. (1994); 80 women; 60+ years; Recruited from seniors' centers in Los Angeles.	One-year intervention study. Two groups: 42 exercise, 38 control. Exercise: program of stand-up, step-up activity; 1-hour sessions, 3 days/week; control: 1 hr./week education. 26% drop-out, 2 deaths. Measured annual fall rate, annual injury rate.	(+) 36% of exercise group and 45% of control group experienced falls in 1 year. 3 serious injuries in controls, no serious injuries in exercisers.
Hornbrook et al. (1994); 3,182 older adults; avg. age = 73.4; 63% female; ambulatory HMO members, independent living.	23-month intervention study. Two groups: exercise = 1,611; control = 1,571. Home risk factor assessment; instruction and manual support for exercises in the home. Walking program 3 times/week walking on one's own; individual exercise program duration and frequency were not reported. 75% of target population was located; of those 51% agreed to participate. Measured self-reported and self-recorded falls on a monthly calender.	(+) Fall rates were lower among exercisers compared to controls. Controls fell 2,084 times while exercise participants fell 1,730 times. The odds of an intervention subject falling was .85 compared to a control participant. Men were less likely to fall and receive injury with falls. Older women may be at more risk of injury in exercise settings which attenuates the positive results of exercise. Survival analysis for injury falls showed no differences.

(Continued)

Table 2-14
(*Continued*)

Researchers and sample	Design, treatment, and measures	Findings
Reinsch et al. (1992); 230 older adults; 60+ years. Recruited from seniors' centers in Los Angeles and Orange County.	One-year intervention study. Four groups: Exercise (stand-up, step-up); Cognitive/behavioral; Exercise and Cog./Behav.; Control. One hr./week. Dropout = 20%, more of the dropouts were previous fallers than were the adherers. Measured self-reported falls; self-reported injury severity on a scale of 7.	(−) No significant differences between groups in time to first fall. 38.6% of the sample suffered at least one fall, but only 7.8% led to a serious injury. Balance, strength and fear of falling did not significantly change. (+) Balance improved in both exercise groups and declined in both non-exercise groups.

who condition strenuously for competition may expect to acquire frequent injuries, some of which may last for years. There is some evidence to suggest that elderly women are more susceptible than men to musculoskeletal injury. The early weeks of initiating activity are a time of injury risk.

Discussion of the Evidence

The potential for injury is often raised as a concern when older adults engage in adventurous or strenuous physical activities. Knowing the actual risks for older people of engaging in various physical activities is valuable in assisting the elderly in making low-risk choices for leisure-time pursuits and for taking steps to reduce risk of injury in work settings.[2]

Aerobic exercise and more vigorous forms of physical activity are the main focus of injury research. Injury which occurs in stretching and strengthening activities needs more attention and needs to be addressed according to the health status of the individuals participating and the nature of the activity. For example, Fuller and Winters (1993), in a study of osteoarthritic aged females, reported that loading forces for side-kick and back-kickleg tasks are somewhat excessive.

---

[2] A number of injury studies have been related to falls in the elderly and these are addressed in the section Falls Outcomes Section (p. 82).

Table 2-15
Falls Outcomes: Correlational and Epidemiological Studies

Researchers and sample	Measures	Findings
Arfken et al. (1994); 875 older adults 65+, Community-dwelling elderly; gender-age stratified sample from St. Louis Older Adult and Information System. Followed for one year.	Visual acuity (Rosenbaum card); difficulty reading; difficulty viewing TV; self-rated vision; bumping into objects. Falls/year; recurrent falls/year.	(+) Bumping into objects predicted falling and recurrent falling. (−) Poor vision did not play a significant role in predicting fallers.
Connell (1993); 28 elderly nursing home residents identified by staff as at-risk of falling. Followed for 2 months.	24-hour video monitoring using a motion-activated camera. Descriptive analysis of the environmental and behavioral factors leading to a fall.	(+) Three broad patterns of falls causation: Multi-tasking, excessive demands in the environment such as changes in light, and inappropriate transfer techniques for current state of health. Researchers concluded that mobile elderly are at risk and interventions should focus on safer ambulation techniques.
Topper et al. (1993); 83 women; 17 men; avg. age = 83 years. Volunteers recruited from 2 self-care residences. Followed one year; 4 deaths without falling; 2 subjects not available at follow-up.	Postural Sway (blind folded posturography); Tinetti Balance & Gait Scale. Number of falls in 1 year. Classifications faller or non-faller.	59 of 100 subjects were fallers; 23 of the fallers were recurrent for a total of 102 falls. (+) Postural sway score predicted fallers versus non-fallers. (−) Other measures not predictive.

(*Continued*)

Table 2-15
(*Continued*)

Researchers and sample	Measures	Findings
O'Loughlin et al. (1993); 409 subjects, 65 years and older. Community-dwelling older adults in Montreal, Canada. Followed 18 months. May 1987 to October 1988. 90% completion rate.	Physical activity, dizziness; alcohol consumption, health status, mobility and medications; social and demographic factors. Incidence rate for falls.	29% of the subjects fell in the follow-up period. (+) Multivariate analyses showed dizziness and frequent physical activity doubled fall risk. Having trouble walking 400 m. (IRR = 1.6) and having trouble bending down (IRR = 1.4) also increased risk of falling. However, protective factors were having diversity in physical activities (IRR = 0.6).
Fleming and Pendergast (1993); 76 women; 19 men; avg. age = 85 years. Adult care facility residents requiring custodial care. Followed 3 years. Deaths were not reported in the study.	Fall location, precipitating activity, hazard, time of occurrence. Peak fall frequency.	(+) Peak fall frequency coincided with periods of activity such as night time toileting. Physical condition and environmental hazards were primary factors in falls. Specific physical activities were implicated in only 7.9% of the falls.
Nevitt et al. (1991); 325; aged 60+; 20% > 80 years. Community-dwelling persons who were ambulatory and who had fallen in the past year. Weekly phone follow-up for one year. Follow-up contacts were 99% complete.	Grip strength, reaction time, circumstances for each fall, falls history. Risk of major injury.	(+) Multivariate analysis revealed that minor injuries were predicted by slower reaction time, decreased grip strength, use of arm support on stairs or steps and when turning around or reaching. Major injuries were higher in persons who had previously fallen with fracture outcomes.

(*Continued*)

Table 2-15
(Continued)

Researchers and sample	Measures	Findings
Speechly and Tinetti (1991); 336 adults 75 years and older. Frail = 77; Transition = 182; Vigorous = 87. Sample subset of Yale Health and Aging Project; able to walk unassisted; independent living in seniors' residences. One year of follow-up after normal activity patterns.	Falls frequency, symptoms, disability, dizziness, mobility, fear of falling, falls history, hearing and vision, sitting to standing blood pressure change, balance and gait assessment. Telephone calls every 2 months to collect falls data; falls from car accidents, acute health problems excluded.	(+) One-year incidence of falling at least once was highest in the frail group (52%) and lowest in the vigorous group (17%). (+) Serious injury was more likely to occur from falls in the vigorous group (22%); 6% serious injury from falls in frail group. 53% of vigorous adults and only 10% of frail adults walked regularly for exercise; 100% of the frail adults and 32% of vigorous adults did no other form of exercise.
Teno et al. (1990); 736 ages 65 to 99 (avg. age = 76.5); 68% female. 10% probability sample of Medicare beneficiaries residing at home in a northeast United States city. Followed 11 months, 35 deaths; 61 refusals for re-interview; 11 were institutionalized, 21 lost to follow-up; 7 lost for misc. reasons.	Walking for exercise less than once/week; Does not engage in sport; Leaves house less than 1 day/week. Measured number of stumbles in the past month. Reported falls in the past 11 months.	(+) Walking less than once per week led to increased relative falls risk of 1.2 while not leaving the house each week led to RR of 1.9. Multiple stumbles in the past month were associated with increased risk of falling in the next year (relative risk of 2.3).

It could be argued that "kicks" should be replaced with more controlled "lifts" in leg exercise for *any* age group. However, it is necessary for researchers and practitioners to be clear that a minority of individuals with health problems may be more susceptible to injury than the average population. Activities which are contraindicated for one group may not be for another. Also injury outcomes are

Table 2-16
Injury Outcomes: Intervention and Comparative Studies

Researchers and sample	Design, treatment, and measures	Findings
Kallinen and Alen (1994); 97 men, ages 70 to 81. Finnish male athletes who were still competitively active; convenience self-selected sample.	10-year retrospective survey data on two types of elderly athletes comparing endurance vs. strength/ power athletes. Varied with involvement in competitive training; many had training diaries as documented evidence. One point in time survey. Measured injury rates during the past 10 years; mechanism and nature of injuries; contributory factors, treatment, healing time, permanent disabilities.	(+) Over 10 years, 81% reported at least 1 sport injury (62% acute, 38% overuse). 75% of athletes had lower extremity injuries; 20% of athletes had knee injury, 19% had foot/ankle injury. Upper extremities most vulnerable to overuse injury; lower extremity more vulnerable to acute sprains. Endurance athletes had more lower limb and joint injury; strength athletes had more muscle and sprain injuries. About 20% of injuries lasted several years; 15% healed within one week.
MacRae et al. (1994); 80 women, 60 and older (avg. age = 72). Community-dwelling older women recruited from seniors' centers in Los Angeles.	One-year intervention study. Two groups: 42 exercise group; 38 attention control group. Exercise: One year low-intensity exercise program using 5 stand-ups from a chair and 5 step-ups onto a step. 3 days/week; 4 sets of 10 repetitions; Attention control: met 1 hour a week. 26% attrition as 21 of the 80 women failed to complete the study (declines in health status, change in work status; death). Measured faller status and severity of injury associated with a fall.	(+) 36% of the exercise group experienced a fall compared to 45% of the control group. None of the exercise group fallers suffered an injury that required medical attention compared with 21% of fallers in the control group. Control group declined significantly in isometric strength of the knee extensors and ankle dorsiflexors while the exercise group did not change significantly.

(Continued)

Table 2-16
(*Continued*)

Researchers and sample	Design, treatment, and measures	Findings
Carroll et al. (1992); 31 males; 37 females; ages 60 to 79. Healthy, sedentary volunteers who were screened by telephone for hypertension, no major diseases.	26-week intervention study. Moderate or high-intensity uphill treadmill walking, 3 times/week; 50% to 80% MaxHR. Adherence was 94.4% for controls, 87.5% for moderate group, and 94.4% for high-intensity group. Measured number and types of injuries related to aerobic treadmill testing and training in walking; VO_2 max (aerobic capacity).	(+) Incidence of injury during walking training was 14%. Low injury rate accompanied by a significant increase in aerobic fitness (16.5% in moderate training group, 23.8% in high-intensity training group). Six of seven injuries occurred in women in the early stages of training when intensity was low. Conclusion: uphill treadmill walking leads to aerobic fitness gains; older women may need to progress slowly to avoid lower limb injury.
Reinsch et al. (1992); 230 adults ages 60 and over. Orange County and Los Angeles County adults from 16 seniors' centers invited to participate in "Senior Body Program."	One-year intervention study. Stand-up, step-up procedure onto a 6-inch stepping stool. Exercise protocol not clear, seems to be up to 1 hour of exercise, 3 times/ week for 1 year; no intensity level assessed. $5.00 monthly honorarium and a wristwatch to keep diary; attrition rate = 20%. Measured fall rates and level of injury.	(−) The program did not make any significant changes to falls or injury outcomes. The researchers felt that the exercise program may not have been intense and regular enough to elicit change. 82% of the falls resulted in low-level injuries (not requiring medical attention).

(*Continued*)

Table 2-16
(Continued)

Researchers and sample	Design, treatment, and measures	Findings
King et al. (1991); 160 women, 197 men, ages 50 to 65. Recruited using telephone random-digit-dialing; Northern California community dwellers who were sedentary and free of cardiac disease.	12-month intervention study. Randomly assigned to four programs of exercise: group low- and high-intensity; at-home low- and high-intensity. High-intensity was 3 × 40-min endurance sessions at 73% to 88% of peak treadmill HR. Lower intensity exercise was 5 × 30 min at 60% to 73% peak HR. Adherence was significantly better for the home-based exercise program (78.7% vs. 75% group-based). Measured exercise-related cardiac events and injuries.	(−) Sprains and fractures were few and were similar across all four intervention groups. Sprains ranged from 3%–10% in each group; fractures of fingers, toes and wrists ranged from 0%–3% in each group (approx. 40 subjects per group). The control group had 0 fractures and 4% sprains. No cardiac events occurred.
Pollock et al. (1991); 25 men, 32 women, ages 70 to 79. Telephone recruitment with some health exclusion.	26 weeks of training intervention study. Randomly assigned to walk-jog program, strength program, or control group. Adherence to training was 87%. Measured exercise-related injuries and comparison across strength and aerobic activities.	(−) One Repetition-Maximum (1-RM) strength testing resulted in 11 injuries (19.3%); while strength training resulted in only 2 injuries (8.7%). Walking training resulted in 1 injury (4.8%). Jogging resulted in injuries in all 6 women and 2 of the 8 men. Because of injuries during 1-RM testing and jogging, caution was advised for these activities.

very much related to the type of sport or activity and its movement requirements (Kallinen & Alen, 1994).

The FIC-SIT trials, a promising research program, was described by Ory et al. (1993). A set of eight different clinical trials concerning physical frailty and injuries in later life, will provide a common database among the eight major sites, with randomized control designs, national representation, and a variety of intervention procedures.

Footwear as a potential factor leading to injuries has not been examined (Ting, 1991). Runners may be particularly vulnerable to inadequate foot protection and cushion against leg strike impact. Some scientists suggest that the very act of being ambulatory puts people at risk of injury, namely fall injury, while others blame lack of exercise on falls injuries (Svanstrom, 1990). The challenge for the application of research to practice for injury prevention requires that "the preventive strategies must strike a balance between the achievement of functional autonomy and patient safety" (Mayo et al., 1993).

Occupational injuries from job-related physical activity are usually treated with physical therapy which involves forms of exercise to bring about strength and mobility improvements. Thus exercise interventions ironically become the solution for injuries caused by being active. It makes intuitive sense that physical deficiencies derived from sedentary living can lead to injury, but it is also true that people do put themselves at risk of injury in certain forms of physical activity. The type of activity does seem to have a significant bearing on injury rate, especially for women. Low-impact, shorter-distance, and submaximal efforts such as walking are recommended in several studies in order to reap the benefits of physical activity with minimal risk of injury.

Chapter 3

Specific Disease Prevention and Management Outcomes

ALZHEIMER'S DISEASE, SENILITY, AND DEMENTIA OUTCOMES

Summary

The level of evidence that exercising adults may reduce the risk for some forms of senile dementia is positive but **weak**. Very little research has been conducted regarding the effects of exercise on the cognitively impaired elderly. The literature suggests that physical activity can help to lessen the complications associated with Alzheimer's disease, but no research has indicated a direct link between physical activity and the chances of developing senile dementia or slowing down its progress. Yet there is some indirect indication that such a link may exist. For example, people who maintain a physically active lifestyle also preserve higher levels of cognitive functioning (see Blumenthal et al., 1991, and the Cognitive Outcomes section of this book). Just as physical activity improves cardiovascular functioning, it also may reduce the risk of strokes, and thereby the risk of multiple infarct dementia. However, these theoretical relationships need to be corroborated by empirical research.

Research in this area needs to separate the effects of exercise from the effects of other potential explanations such as social attention and social interaction. Pre and post comparisons and control groups would be useful for comparing different types of interventions. Also necessary is a focus on a variety of possible outcomes of exercise interventions, including medical, behavioral, social, and psychological changes related to dementia.

Discussion of the Evidence

A few studies investigating the relationship between physical activity and senile dementia were reviewed by Bonner and O'Brien Cousins (1996). In the 1970s, three carefully controlled intervention studies were conducted to examine the effect of exercise on mentally disturbed elderly, but the results were mixed. One study (Clark et al., 1975) did not find any statistically significant effects. The other two studies (Powell, 1974; Stamford et al., 1974) found positive effects on some measures of cognitive functioning.

Mace (1987) found that physical activity decreased the occurrence of uncontrolled, repetitive behavior such as wandering, pulling at clothing, and making repetitive noises. These behaviors, while common among cognitively impaired elders, may be ameliorated with regular physical activity such as walking. In another study, a three times a week, nine-week musical exercise program was administered to Alzheimer's patients who exhibited behaviors such as spitting, hitting, and scratching. At the end of the nine weeks, there was an increased ability on the part of the participating patients to follow directions and to engage in social interaction (Beck et al., 1992).

Friedman and Tappen (1991) compared the effect of a walking/conversation intervention to a conversation-only condition on communication skills of Alzheimer's patients. They found that the walking group improved their communication significantly while the conversation-only group did not improve at all. The results of this study suggested that there is promise in the use of exercise in the treatment and care of elderly patients, but further research is needed. Table 3-1 presents findings from intervention studies. No correlational studies are reported.

CORONARY HEART DISEASE OUTCOMES

Summary

The level of evidence for coronary heart disease (CHD) outcomes is **acceptable**. CHD refers to diseases of the heart and blood vessels that supply the heart, and it is currently one of the leading causes of death in North America. Risk of CHD increases with age, and incidence of CHD may be on the rise in elderly populations (Bild et al., 1993).

There have been several risk factors associated with CHD. Modifiable risks include hypertension, stress, tobacco smoking, elevated blood fat and cholesterol levels, physical inactivity, and obesity.

These risk factors are listed as primary by the American Heart Association and have a high association with CHD. Risks that cannot be controlled include

Table 3-1
Alzheimer's and Dementias Outcomes: Intervention and Comparison Studies

Researchers and sample	Design, treatment, and measures	Findings
Friedman and Tappen (1991); 13 females, 17 males; ages 60 to 87 (avg. age = 72.8); diagnosed with probable Alzheimer's according to NINCDS-ADRDA criteria.	10-week intervention study. Random assignment to groups (15 treatment, 15 control). Treatment: One-on-one conversation while walking for 30 min. Control: one-on-one conversation only (30 min.). 3 times/week, no dropouts reported. Communication Measures: Cognitively Impaired Scale (CAS), Communication Observation Scale for the Cognitively Impaired (COS).	(+) Walking group increased significantly more on communication skill (COS) than conversation only group. (+ n.s.) Similar pattern on CAS, but did not reach significance.
Meddaugh (1987); 4 females, 5 males; avg. age = 75. Nursing home; confused, abusive behavior; dependent in activities of daily living. Staff hypothesized that patients would not be able to follow instructions to do the exercises.	9-week intervention study. Exercise to music, with positive reinforcement of desired behaviors. Duration not specified; 3 times/week. Participation an average of 1.5 times per week. Measures: descriptions of: social interactions, willingness to try exercises, ability to do exercises, "acceptable" behavior, "unacceptable" behavior.	(+) Three patients were able to do all the exercises; one patient decreased verbal swearing; a few talked to each other or smiled from time to time; staff morale improved; program was continued after the study.

aging, heredity, and gender. Other factors associated with CHD include electro-cardiogram abnormalities, glucose intolerance, male pattern baldness, diabetes mellitus, disabilities, and diet. The majority of research tends to support a positive role for physical activity in prevention and/or reduction of CHD risk factors in the elderly. Prior chronic physical activity or athleticism may not guard against CHD unless physical activity patterns are maintained over the life span. Incidence of CHD increases after age 35 among men and after menopause among women (50+).

Discussion of the Evidence

Aging is associated with a decline of about 10% per decade in cardiovascular function, with maximum heart rate decreasing as a result of neural, hormonal, and functional changes. Stroke volume is reduced mainly because of a decrease in myocardial contractility and blood flow to the heart also falls. This latter finding is due to a general atherosclerotic condition that includes a decrease in vessel elasticity, and in the cross-sectional area of the lumen of the coronary arteries and other vessels. These changes are accompanied by an increase in blood pressure (hypertension) with age. Associated with these age-related cardiovascular changes are decreases in muscle strength, lean body mass, pulmonary lung function, and maximal oxygen consumption, as well as a decline in some aspects of neurological functioning.

The result of this multitude of factors is an increase in the risk of CHD with aging. However, lower than expected rates for CHD have been shown in subjects ages 85 years and older, especially males (Bild et al., 1993). As suggested by those authors, this may have been due to a sample or mortality selection bias, or to a plateau in CHD prevalence with elderly subjects.

Prior athleticism does not seem to affect CHD risk factors (Brill et al., 1989). However, Hein et al. (1994) reported that there was a lower risk of ischemic heart disease (IHD) in men who were physically active upon reaching middle age and who *continued* to be active. Furthermore, Hein et al. showed that CHD risk doubled in men ages 50 to 59 when they initiated an active lifestyle after years of being sedentary, suggesting that prescribing sudden activity for sedentary middle-age men must be done with medical clearance and monitoring.

Physical activity has generally been associated with an improvement in risk factors associated with CHD (Tuomilehto et al., 1987; Darga et al., 1989; Leveille et al., 1993; Hein et al., 1994). Physical activity in combination with a healthy diet has also been shown to reduce circulating fats, cholesterol, and low-density lipoproteins, and to increase high-density lipoproteins in the elderly (Darga et al., 1989; Barnard, 1991; Caspersen et al., 1991; Singh et al., 1993; Puggaard et al., 1994). Systemic blood pressure can be lowered with increased physical activity in the aged, provided the exercise stimulus is sufficient (see Hypertension section). Increased physical activity can lower stress and enhance well-being.

Increased levels of blood fats or serum lipids (cholesterol, triglycerides, and lipoproteins, especially low-density lipoprotein) have been associated with CHD in the elderly and may be considered independent risk factors (Kannel & Vokonas, 1986; Aronow et al., 1986, 1989; Castelli et al., 1989; Wong et al., 1990; Rubin et al., 1990). Aronow and Ahn (1994) suggested that total cholesterol, low-density lipoproteins (LDL), and high-density lipoproteins (HDL) were independent risk factors in elderly men and women. For instance, total cholesterol may be normal but HDL may be low in CHD subjects.

However, some research in previously sedentary elderly women failed to show an improvement in serum lipid or lipoprotein profiles after 12 weeks of moderate endurance training (Nieman et al., 1993). Caution is needed in evaluating serum lipids as the circulating levels can fluctuate because of seasonal rhythm, dietary factors, and activity patterns (Puggaard et al., 1994).

Participating in physical activity may enhance glucose tolerance in the elderly as a result of increased insulin sensitivity of skeletal muscle (Richter & Galbo, 1986), though other research has not had similar results (Seals et al., 1984b; Puggaard et al., 1994). Further research into the role of physical activity in glucose tolerance in the elderly is needed. Improved nutrition and diet can reduce glucose intolerance and probably help control blood glucose levels in patients with diabetes mellitus. Tables 3-2 and 3-3 address intervention and comparative and correlational and epidemiological studies, respectively.

BONE HEALTH AND OSTEOPOROSIS OUTCOMES

Summary

The level of evidence for bone health and osteoporosis outcomes is **acceptable**. Osteoporosis "is a condition in which the amount of bone tissue is so low that the bones easily fracture in response to minimal force" (Aloia, 1989). Osteoporosis results when the body has not obtained an adequate amount of mineral (calcium mostly) from the environment and when the mechanical load is insufficient for development of new bone as a result of physical inactivity. This lack of bone density can reach a critical level in the elderly which leaves the individual susceptible to bone damage because of what are normally incidental structural impacts.

Exercise across the life span is important in both the development and maintenance of bone density. Vigorous forms of exercise are critical at adolescence, especially for females, for the initial creation of optimal bone mass. It is essential that weight-bearing exercise accompany later life stages, for women especially, for maintaining bone mass. Weight-bearing or resistance-loaded exercise is more effective than non-loaded exercise in developing bone mass. This raises the question of which specific forms of exercise are most valuable to older adults for maintaining bone mass.

Deconditioning (as a result of illness or the cessation of exercise) reverses the gains made in bone strength. Long-term benefits are only retained if exercise

Table 3-2
Coronary Heart Disease Outcomes: Intervention and Comparative Studies

Researchers and sample	Design, treatment, and measures	Findings
Puggaard et al. (1994); 59 men and women; avg. age = 67; volunteers, healthy.	5-month intervention study, no control. 45 minutes of gymnastics and dancing or 25 minutes of swimming; 2 sessions per week at a relative workload of 58% to 65% of maxHR, 91% attendance rate. Measures: variety of fitness tests, serum lipids, BP, dietary habits.	(+) Significant decrease in LDL and increase in HDL. (−) No change in triglycerides, or total cholesterol. (+) General decrease in CHD risk.
Nieman et al. (1993); 42 older women; sedentary, healthy volunteers in training competing in endurance sports; avgerage 11 years training.	12-week intervention study. Two groups: 32 untrained (avg. age = 71); 10 trained (avg. age = 73.4). Brisk walking and calisthenics for 30 to 40 minutes per session; 5 days a week at 60% of heart rate reserve. Measured serum lipid profile and a variety of other measures.	(+) Highly trained group had significantly higher HDL-C and lower triglycerides.
Singh et al. (1993); 621 patients. Men and women.	Multiple-stage intervention study. Randomly assigned to intervention or control group. Diet and exercise program (Indian Diet Heart Study). Initial 3 weeks observation, followed by 16-week diet, then an 8-week diet and exercise. Measured serum lipids, BP, diet profile, CHD risk factors.	(+) A significant decrease in total cholesterol, LDL-C triglycerides, fasting blood glucose, blood pressure, and CHD risk factors in the intervention group.

(Continued)

Table 3-2
(*Continued*)

Researchers and sample	Design, treatment, and measures	Findings
Takeshima et al. (1993); 12 males, 11 females, ages 60 to 79 (avg. age = 69). Healthy volunteers, no past training.	12-week intervention study. Endurance training: 30 min recreational and 30 min cycling. 3 times/ week at lactate threshold intensity. Serum lipids and fitness variables measured.	(+) Significant decreases in total cholesterol and triglycerides. (−) No change in HDL-C, LDL-C, or atherogenic index.
Barnard (1991); 2,685 males (avg. age = 56.5) and 1,902 females (avg. age = 55.6). Ages 20 to 88 males, 20 to 92 females. Participants in Pritikin Center program; 33% had CHD, 43% hypertension, 16% diabetes mellitus.	Intervention study of 21 days of a diet and exercise regime. Daily aerobic exercise. Serum lipid profile assessed.	(+) Significant improvement in all serum lipid blood variables except the total cholesterol to HDL ratio in female subjects.

resumes in a short period of time and is maintained. Also, bone remineralization capability appears to be dependent on initial bone mass and training intensity. This suggests that people with extremely low initial bone mass may have more to gain through exercise than those with near adequate bone density, but the former may never attain the same degree of bone density.

While it may be difficult for seniors to *increase* their bone mass through participation in exercise, exercise does maintain bone and slow the rate of bone loss which accompanies aging.

Discussion of the Evidence

Increasingly research has identified that the early years of development of an individual are a critical time in maximizing potential bone mass (for a review, see Drinkwater, 1994). For maximal gains, the period from the teen years through age 30 to 40 years is essential in creating a high bone density which will last the life span. The higher the peak bone mass obtained and maintained, the less likely that, with the declines of aging, an individual will enter the critically low bone density

Table 3-3
Coronary Heart Disease Outcomes: Correlational and Epidemiological Studies

Researchers and sample	Measures	Findings
Hein et al. (1994); 2,894 men, avg. age = 63. 6-year follow-up to Copenhagen male study; 75% survival rate.	Two groups: less than 4 hrs/week of physical activity and greater than 4 hrs/week of activity. Measured lifestyle and CHD risk factors.	(+) Lowest rate of ischemic heart disease was found in the active men.
Caspersen et al. (1991); 863 men., 65 to 84 years old. Zutphen Study investigating CHD risk and physical activity. 1985 survey and examination procedure. 74.2 % of the original sample participated.	Physical activity patterns and CHD risk factors. Physical activity questionnaire, serum lipids, BP, lifestyle questionnaire.	(+) Total weekly physical activity and specific activities such as walking were positively associated with lower cholesterol and systolic blood pressure.

level associated with osteoporosis. Cheng et al. (1993) found significant differences in bone mineral density (BMD) according to the physical activity histories of their subjects (for men when they were under 20, and when women were between the ages of 20 and 49). Similar results are shown by Ballard et al. (1990) and Suominen and Rahkila (1991), where an active involvement in exercise across the life span was associated with greater bone densities later in life.

Research has found conflicting evidence regarding seniors' capacity to add bone mass to their skeletal systems at an advanced age. Results from Greendale et al. (1993) and Martin and Notelowitz (1993) failed to find any significant change in bone densities between exercisers and sedentary subjects. While more intense exercise can increase bone mass slightly, evidence suggests that moderate weight-bearing exercise may play an integral role in minimizing the rate of bone loss, thus delaying the possibility of osteoporosis (Hatori et al., 1993; Grove & Londeree, 1992). As with many other body systems, the greatest benefits seem to be for those individuals who have a low bone density to begin with. It is they who stand to gain the greatest benefit from exercise. Some researchers suggest that remineralization of bone may be more effective when exercise is used in combination with calcium supplementation and/or estrogen or testosterone therapy.

Table 3-4
Osteoporosis Outcomes: Intervention and Comparative Studies

Researchers and sample	Design, treatment, and measures	Findings
Greendale et al. (1993); 30 women, 6 men; ages 58 to 80; volunteers from senior center. Subjects excluded for inability to complete questionnaire independently, heart problems, several other physical disorders.	20-week intervention study. Randomized control study with 2 groups: 19 exercisers, 17 controls. Exercise group wore weighted vests for 2 weeks, then wore them at home at their own discretion. Both groups met for 1 hour each week for 20 weeks. Discussion (control) group was led by experts on health education. Five dropped out. Measured bone mineral density (BMD) of L2-L4 vertebral bodies with an X-ray densitometer.	(+ n.s.) There was a small increase in BMD for exercise subjects and a small decline in BMD for control subjects. Results did not reach significance (perhaps due to small sample size).
Hatori et al. (1993); 33 women. Ages 45 to 67. All postmenopausal women.	7-month intervention study. Randomized control study, 3 groups: High-Intensity Exercise (about 110% of max HR at aerobic threshold); Moderate-Intensity Exercise (about 90% of maxHR at the aerobic threshold); control group. Subjects walked at designated intensity for 30 min, 3 times/week. 2 dropouts. Measured bone mineral density (BMD) of lumbar spine (L2-L4) by dual-energy X-ray absorptiometry.	(+) While there was a small decrease in BMD for the control and moderate-intensity groups, there was a small but significant increase in BMD for high-intensity participants.

(*Continued*)

Table 3-4
(*Continued*)

Researchers and sample	Design, treatment, and measures	Findings
Martin and Notelovitz (1993); 55 women, average age 58. All subjects at least 12 mos. post-menopausal; Caucasian, non-smoking, no medication interfering in calcium metabolism, no strength or aerobic training.	One-year randomized control study with 3 groups: Exercise 30 min or 45 min; control. All subjects took calcium supplements. Exercise training 3 times/week. Intensity: 70% to 85% of maxHR on a treadmill. Measured BMD by dual-energy photon absorptiometry (lumbar), single-energy photon absorptiometry for forearm.	(−) There were no significant differences in either lumbar or forearm BMDs between any of the groups.
Grove and Londeree (1992); 15 women, ages 49 to 64. Healthy, early post-menopausal, sedentary, Caucasian.	One-year randomized control study, 3 groups: high- or low-impact exercise, controls. Exercise: 15–20 min warmup, 20 min supervised exercise (high or low impact), 15 min cool down. BMD measure: dual photon absorptiometry on the vertebrae (L2-L4).	(+) The non-exercising group showed significant decline in BMD; exercising groups maintained BMD. There was no significant difference between exercise groups.
Lau et al. (1992); 50 Chinese women, ages 62 to 92 years. Women with metabolic bone disease, history of hip fracture, or blood creatinine levels over 125 umol/l excluded from study.	10-month intervention study. Randomized control study with 4 groups: Calcium supplement (800 mg/day); Load-bearing exercise and placebo tablet; Load-bearing exercise and calcium supp.; Placebo control. Exercise groups: 100 step-ups, 15 min submax exercise; BMD measured at (femoral neck, Ward's triangle, and intertrochanteric area) and the L2–L4 level of the spine.	(+) There was a significant combined effect of exercise and calcium on femoral neck bone mass. (−) Exercise alone had no effect on bone loss at any site. Significant increase in BMD at Ward's triangle and intertrochanteric subjects on calcium supp; no significant change at the femoral neck.

(*Continued*)

Table 3-4

(*Continued*)

Researchers and sample	Design, treatment, and measures	Findings
Nelson et al. (1991); 36 women, avg. age 60.2 years, with none over age 70. Post-menopausal Caucasian women; not involved in exercise, weighed < 130% of ideal body weight, and were not taking estrogen.	One-year intervention study. Exercise and control groups (non-random, self-selected). Subjects also randomly assigned to a calcium supplement or placebo group. Exercise: supervised walk for 50 min, 4 times/week. After 4 weeks, wore weight belts. Subjects exercised at 70%–85% of Max HR. Measured bone density by hydrostatic weighing; BMD by single-photon absorptiometry.	(+) Exercise was determined to have a significant positive effect on the BMD of trabecular bone of the spine, and on femoral bone density.
Rikli and McManis (1990); 31 women; ages 57 to 83; post-menopausal.	10-month intervention study. Three groups: General exercise; General exercise plus weight training; Control. General exercise: warm-up, cool down, 20–30 of large muscle aerobic activity at 60%–70% of maxHR. Weight training: 20 min resistance training of upper body. Three times/week. Measured BMC by single-photon bone densitometer.	(+) There were significant differences between exercise and control groups. The exercise group experienced an increase in bone mineral content (BMC) while the control group experienced a loss of BMC. No significant differences were found between the two exercise groups.
Blumenthal et al. (1989); 51 women; 50 men; ages 60 to 83 (avg. age = 67); healthy but sedentary volunteers.	4-month intervention study. Randomly assigned to 3 groups: aerobic exercise; yoga; wait list. Aerobic: 3 times/week, 30 min; Yoga: 60 min, 2 times/week, 4 months. Measured bone density by bone densitometer. BMC from distal radius of non-dominant arm.	(+) For subjects at risk for bone fracture (low BMD), there was an increase in BMD with exercise. (−) No significant effect for those with 'healthy' BMDs.

Table 3-5

Osteoporosis Outcomes: Correlational and Epidemiological Studies

Researchers and sample	Measures	Findings
Krall and Dawson-Hughes (1994); 239 Caucasian women, ages 42 to 72; at least two years post-menopausal, in good health. Followed for 1 year; 37 dropouts.	Self-reported sports and leisure activities, number of miles walked per week, historical physical activity patterns. BMD measured by dual-energy absorptiometry on the spine (L2-L4).	(+) Women who walked more than 7.5 miles/ week had higher mean bone density of the trunk and whole body than women who walked less than 1 mile/week. Walking also slowed the rate of bone loss from the legs.
Cheng et al. (1993); 188 women, 103 men; all 75 years old; born in 1914 in Jyvaskyla, Finland. No subject excluded on the basis of disease; cross-sectional study.	Self-reported physical activity, diet, smoking and drinking habits, health, socioeconomic status, marital status. BMD measured by single-energy photon absorption.	(+) BMD was higher in men with moderate levels of physical activity than in those with low activity. BMD correlated significantly with physical activity before age 20 and during age 75 in men and during the age period 20–49 in women. Men had 36% higher BMD than women, and were still 17% higher when corrected for bone size.
Rutherford and Jones (1992); 216 women, ages 21–82. 185 subjects over 40, 140 subjects over 50. Healthy British Caucasian women. None suffering from any endocrine or metabolic disorder, systemic illness, or bone or muscle disease. One session.	Self-reported medical, menstrual, and physical activity history. Computerized tomography scans: mid-shaft and distal femur. Spine density measured using dual-energy X-ray absorptiometry (L1-L4).	(+) Significant positive relationship between quadricep strength and bone mass at all three sites. (−) However, with age kept constant, current physical activity levels did not correlate with any of the muscle or bone indices.

(Continued)

Table 3-5
(*Continued*)

Researchers and sample	Measures	Findings
Suominen and Rahkila (1991); 139 men, ages 70 to 81. Veteran members of Finnish sports organizations (endurance, strength-trained, speed trained); control group randomly selected from population.	Cross-sectional study, one time only data collection. Self-reported exercise and dietary habits. BMD measured by single-energy photon absorption.	(+) BMD was significantly higher for endurance and speed trained athletes than controls. Although strength-trained athletes had higher mean values than controls, this did not reach significance.
Ballard et al. (1990); 91 women; ages 50 to 68. Subjects were community volunteers with divergent levels of physical activity and a mixture of those who had and had not had estrogen therapy.	One data collection session. Self-reported dietary records, physical activity, gynecological survey, medical history. Bone mass measured with bone densitometer. Physical condition measured by submaximal exercise test on treadmill (modified Balke treadmill protocol) to determine work capacity in METs.	(+) High physical activity subjects had significantly higher BMC than low physical activity subjects. Estrogen therapy subjects had higher bone mass than non-estrogen therapy subjects.

Comprehensive research is needed to determine which forms of physical activity make the best contribution to bone density for older adults. What is the contribution of aquatic resistance exercise versus land exercise programs? How much is lost if walking is done in water versus on land? Is regular walking and activity around the home as good for maintaining bone health as a supervised exercise program (given equal time and intensity)? Is progressive resistance training superior to other forms of loaded exercise? Are there gender differences in the effectiveness, timing, and types of exercise which can retard bone loss? These and other questions need to be answered if practitioners and health promotion consultants are to advise aging adults intelligently on how best to prevent or treat osteoporosis.

ARTHRITIS OUTCOMES

Summary

The level of evidence for the role of physical activity in decreasing the symptoms of osteoarthritis is **indicative**. Osteoarthritis is characterized by the degradation of the articular cartilage, leading to a loss of joint stability, less mobility, and a considerable amount of pain (Moskowitz et al., 1992). Osteoarthritis is the most prevalent chronic condition in persons 65 and older, causing functional impairment, morbidity, and often increased use of health care services. After age 35, osteoarthritis is present in one to two out of three people (Moskowitz et al., 1992). It is the most frequently reported cause of disability among Americans, accounting for 12.3% of all persons with activity limitations (Hampson et al., 1993). Most adults over 65 will encounter the disease in varying degrees.

Contrary to popular opinion, runners and athletes are not prone to osteoarthritis as a result of years of training (Lane et al., 1993; Lane et al., 1990). In the 1990 study, Lane and colleagues matched 34 older runners (average age 59) with 34 same-age sedentary individuals. All subjects underwent a rheumatological examination and roentgenography of hands, spine, and weight-bearing joints before and after two years of follow-up. This study found that a strict running regimen did not induce further developments of osteoarthritis, whereas the disease progressed among the sedentary sample.

The strongest conclusion regarding arthritis and active living outcomes is that light to vigorous levels of physical activity do not exacerbate arthritis and related symptoms (Hannan et al., 1993; Konradsen et al., 1990; Lane et al., 1993; Minor & Brown, 1993). On the contrary, osteoarthritic individuals are likely to increase their problems by reducing activity and thereby increasing synovial thickening, effusion, pain, and joint instability (Hall et al., 1993).

Discussion of the Evidence

A few studies demonstrate that active living can increase function and decrease arthritic pain. Supervised walking among 102 volunteers with chronic osteoarthritis (average age of 69.4 years) led to significant improvements in natural stride length and walking velocity (Petersen et al., 1993). More importantly, the intervention group experienced reduced pain. Kovar et al. (1992) published another aspect of the same study in which the patient education part of the program was examined. Guest speakers discussed the medical aspects of osteoarthritis, barriers to and benefits of exercise, proper walking technique, and how to adhere to a scheduled walking program. After eight weeks, the exercise group showed a definite improvement in knowledge about osteoarthritis and the benefits of exercise, whereas the control group showed none. In addition, the exercisers reported a lower level of pain during the walking test, and they used less medication.

Dexter (1992) studied 110 community-living elderly who were diagnosed with osteoarthritis according to the American College of Rheumatology classification system. All subjects were over age 50 and had impairments ranging from no mobility to slow walking. Dexter assessed the current activity patterns of these adults. About 60% never performed any special exercises for their arthritis, 5.5% did so once a week, and 34.5% did so at least several times a week. Almost 40% had never received medical advice to exercise. Upon observation of the exercisers, many were not performing exercises with proper technique. This study demonstrated a need for physicians to take a stronger advocacy role for exercise and for exercises to be supervised or at least adequately learned.

Water-based exercise has shown the potential to improve both physical and psychological well-being for participants with osteoarthritis. Meyer and Hawley (1994) compared 87 participants with rheumatic disease attending a community-based water exercise program with 174 age- and sex-matched patients attending a rheumatic disease clinic. Clinic patients reported higher pain scores, higher levels of functional disability, more anxiety, more depression, higher severity scores, and lower grip strength than the water exercise participants.

Low-impact activity may be helpful even if self-managed at home (Hampson et al., 1993). In this study, 61 participants of average age 72 from Lane County, Oregon were diagnosed with osteoarthritis for at least one year. Self-report questionnaires were used to document which forms of self-management of osteoarthritis were used by participants on "typical" and "worse than usual" days. More self-management methods were used on worse days, while typical days were accompanied by gentle forms of activity. Of particular interest is the finding that the use of low-impact exercise such as walking, swimming, and range-of-motion exercises was positively correlated with the reduction of osteoarthritis pain. Other studies have also found decreased pain and morning stiffness as a result of physical activity intervention (Allegrante et al., 1993; Minor & Brown, 1993).

Similarly, Green et al. (1993) reported that home exercise was as therapeutic as physiotherapy treatments for osteoarthritis patients. Forty-seven patients (average age 67) were divided randomly into two treatment groups, engaged in either an eight-week home exercise program or an eight-week home exercise program plus hydrotherapy. For the home exercises, each subject was given a written description of five exercises and a log book to fill in twice a day. The hydrotherapy was conducted twice a week by a therapist. Because all patients in both groups showed improvement over the eight-week period, the hydrotherapy could not demonstrate any extra utility. The implication was that without hydrotherapy costs, and relying instead on at-home exercise, reductions in health care would be possible.

The majority of studies represent subjects in later stages of the life span, as the condition is more prevalent in these cohorts. One study found that age was the best predictor of arthritis risk (Lane et al., 1993). However, few researchers evaluate the advantages of active living according to age. More research has been done with women than men, perhaps because of the large numbers of women with arthritis. Another longitudinal study which accommodated the age variable found that older adults with arthritis reported more difficulty walking than those without arthritis, and the percent with difficulty walking increased with age. Table 3-6 summarizes studies addressing the relationship between physical activity and arthritis. Because of the small number of studies reviewed, intervention/comparison and correlational/epidemiological are combined in the one table. Most studies deal with osteoarthritis (OA); some with rheumatoid arthritis (RA).

CHRONIC OBSTRUCTIVE PULMONARY DISEASE OUTCOMES

Summary

The level of evidence for the relationship between physical activity and chronic obstructive pulmonary disease (COPD) is **weak**. COPD includes chronic bronchitis and emphysema and is the fifth leading cause of death (O'Donnell et al., 1993). Previous tobacco use in today's older adults is blamed for the rising morbidity and mortality rates for COPD. In both the United Kingdom and the United States, COPD is the major cause of restricted activity and work incapacity. No therapeutic intervention other than early smoking cessation has been shown to alter the declining pulmonary function and progressive breathlessness of smokers (O'Donnell et al., 1993). It follows that for patients with acute irreversible disease, symptom alleviation is the main therapeutic goal, and thus exercise had been considered an important treatment modality for over 20 years.

Contemporary studies examining the role of exercise training with COPD adults indicate that older adults may obtain less spectacular cardiovascular benefits than younger. However, there have been few clinically controlled studies with elderly COPD adults, and sample sizes for exercise intervention studies have been small. More studies are therefore needed to confirm the effect of exercise training on COPD symptoms (e.g, in the very old, those with co-morbidity, those at different stages of the disease, and those whose COPD is smoking-related versus caused by other factors). Also, the majority of current COPD elderly have been men; research with women is scarce.

Table 3-6
Arthritis Outcomes

Researchers and sample	Treatment and measures	Findings
Stenstrom (1994); 56 female, 13 males; over 70 years (avg. age = 54). Convenience sample, Swedish. R.A. symptoms for 14 years, not treated; 14% dropped out of study.	Followed for 4 years; categorized as low-versus high-frequency exercise; measured joint destruction every two years.	(−) No difference between groups in demographics or disease severity.
Lane et al. (1993); 98 older adults, ages 50 to 72 yrs. Runners in a 50 years plus club.	Two groups: 41 athletes, 57 matched controls. Athletes followed their normal running program; 33 followed up for 5 years. Radiographs used to assess O.A. of knee, hand, and spine.	(−) No significant difference in O.A. between athletes and matched controls. Best predictor of O.A. was older age.
Peterson et al. (1993); 102 older adults with osteoarthritis. Patients with osteoarthritis of the knee.	Two groups: Exercise: 8-week walking and education program. Controls: phoned weekly for education. Measured walking distance, stride length, and speed.	(+) Walking and gait function improved in the intervention group.
Minor and Brown (1993); 120 total O.A. = 80. R.A. = 40. Ages 21 to 83 years. O.A. = 64 years; R.A. = 54 years; 82% female; 95% Caucasian; 30% employed.	Randomly assigned to one of three groups: Aerobic walking program; Aerobic aquatic program; Controls: (stretching exercises). Program ran for 12 weeks, 60 min/session; 3 times/ week. 81% adherence. Measured fitness, arthritis, pain, exercise behavior (a number of measures of each). 3-, 6-, 9-month follow-up.	(+) More active exercise behavior was associated with low pain but only at 18 months; causality is not determined.

(Continued)

Table 3-6
(*Continued*)

Researchers and Sample	Treatment and measures	Findings
Konradsen et al. (1990); 27 Danish men, sedentary controls, matched for height, weight and age.	Two groups: 27 runners, 27 controls. Runners continued as per individual training regime. 90% adherence. Roentgenograph assessment. Arthritis pain and joint measurements.	(−) No difference between runners and controls for symptoms of arthritis.

Discussion of the Evidence

Contemporary research on older adults has found that the exercising COPD elderly can make significant increases in aerobic physiological parameters and fitness performance, although the young-old appear to make more gains than the old-old over 80 (Emery, 1994; Swertz et al., 1990; Toshima et al., 1990; Weaver & Narsavage, 1992). Breathlessness has also been shown to be reduced (O'Donnell et al., 1993).

The beneficial training effects of exercise for COPD sufferers are similar to those of healthy non-COPD adults, but effects in COPD patients are less consistent. Some studies do not identify the specific age group under study. Thus, a good deal of research has been conducted on the benefits of exercise in COPD adults, but it is not clear how much of the data involves older adults. There are few studies which specifically focus on older adult populations.

There is no clear consensus as to whether older patients with COPD uniformly achieve physiological effects from exercise training (O'Donnell et al., 1993). Although some studies have reported positive training effects, others have not. Furthermore, interpretation of results has been confounded by

(a) the paucity of controlled clinical studies;
(b) variation in study populations with respect to disease severity or existence of comorbid conditions;
(c) uncertainty regarding clinical stability of the disease at the outset of training; and
(d) failure to consider subjective outcome parameters such as perceived breathlessness.

Whether aerobic capacity is improved following training in the COPD elderly is controversial. Earlier studies failed to show this. More recent studies using higher levels of training intensity in patients with moderate COPD have shown significant lactate reductions with concomitant reductions in ventilation during exercise. Furthermore, the safety of exercise training among COPD older adults has been demonstrated repeatedly, even in elderly patients with advanced disease and chronic ventilatory failure (Alpert et al., 1975; Belman & Kendregan, 1981; Degre et al., 1974; Paez et al., 1967; Casaburi et al., 1991). Evidence concerning exercise and COPD symptoms is summarized in Table 3-7.

CANCER OUTCOMES

Summary

The level of evidence for the link between physical activity and cancer in older adults is **indicative**. Evidence is rapidly accumulating for an association between elevated risk of several cancers and a sedentary lifestyle. The bulk of research comes from epidemiological studies which attempt to control for possible confounding variables.

The studies presented in Table 3-8 include breast, endometrial, colon, rectal, and renal cell cancers. None of the studies demonstrated a dose response relationship with cancer and physical activity, yet all found some level of statistical significance regarding elevated risk by physical inactivity.

The biological links between cancer and active living are not well understood. For example, Shu et al. (1993) stated that "obesity is a well recognized risk factor for endometrial cancer, but the mechanism is not well understood" (p. 342). Factors contributing to an elevated risk of cancer that may interact with physical activity are diet and body mass index, yet more evidence is required to establish these links clearly. Immune response may play a role, and some evidence indicates that the immune system is strengthened through active living. As the site of the cancer changes, so does the possibility for confounding variables.

The role of age in these relationships is not well addressed. We do not know if active living has a more important role at earlier stages of life, and if late-life exercise can improve prospects for successful treatment in one's older years.

A few studies have concluded that active living is a beneficial process for patients with cancer. Active living makes a number of contributions to quality of life and probably elevates the sense of well-being or control required to live with a disease like cancer. More rehabilitation centers are including active living experiences as part of the healing process.

Table 3-7

Chronic Obstructive Pulmonary Disease Outcomes: Intervention and Comparative Studies

Researchers and sample	Treatment and measures	Findings
Emery (1994); 29 females, 35 males; avg. age = 67.4 (range 53 to 82). Convenience sample of older outpatients in a pulmonary rehab program at Duke University's Center for Living (55% male). No control group.	Small group program for 30 days; 4 hours per session; respiratory therapy plus warm-up floor exercises, 45 min aerobic exercise and Nautilus strength training. Five days per week; no intensity reported. Two females and one male dropped out for unexplained reasons. Measured forced vital capacity (FVC); VO_2max using cycle ergometry; timed 12 min walk for distance.	(+) All subjects showed significant improvement at post-exercise in all 3 aerobic fitness measures with older individuals making significantly less improvement than younger adults of less than 67.5 years. Cardiopulmonary improvement may not increase as rapidly among older-old.
O'Donnell et al. (1993); 36 older adults (avg. age = 66). Clinically stable patients with advanced COPD.	Two age-matched groups: 23 exercisers, 13 controls. Exercise: multi-modality endurance training program, 2–3 hours/session over 8 weeks; 3 times/week; intensity not reported. Measured breathlessness by BDI (Baseline Dyspnea Index), OCD (Oxygen Cost Diagram), and MRC (Medica Research Council) scales.	(+) Compared with controls, the exercise group achieved highly significant reduction in breathlessness.

(Continued)

Table 3-7
(*Continued*)

Researchers and sample	Treatment and measures	Findings
Swerts et al. (1990); 24 men, 3 women. COPD outpatients. No controls.	Eight-week rehabilitation program followed by 12 weeks of either at-home exercise (14 subjects) or same program with supervision (11 subjects). Three times/week; self-paced walking for 30 min, relaxation training for 30 min, cycling for 15 min at 50% to 70% of max heart rate. One patient died; 2 dropped out for unreported reasons. Measures: 12 min walk test; Breathlessness Score (Likert scale); lung function (FVC, FEV); symptom-limited bicycle exercise test.	(+) Measurable improvement in exercise tolerance on the 12 min walk test. A significant improvement in walking distance persisted after 26 and 52 weeks. Adherence rates for the supervised group were superior to the at-home exercise group. (−) This effect of physical training was not accompanied by ventilatory improvements.

Discussion of the Evidence

The majority of this research includes adults in the later stages of the life cycle, though none of the studies are specific to older adults (Mellemgaard et al., 1994; Satariano et al., 1990; Levi et al., 1993). Satariano et al. (1990), in a case control study, examined 900 women to determine whether having breast cancer affects physical activities such as strength and range of motion. They compared results between cases and controls as well as between three age groups from 55 to 84 years old. Cancer patients had significantly poorer function than controls, probably because of health and activity differences.

Several problems plague large-scale studies. Physical activity has been examined through a variety of instruments, yet there remain a lack of standardized acceptable tools. For example, a few studies have used occupational physical activity classifications (Shu et al., 1993; Gerhardson et al., 1990; Mellemgaard et al., 1994). However, the job codes may not apply to less industrialized countries, and they exclude large segments of the population such as retirees and women who work inside the home. Also, occupational activity level may be systematically confounded with other variables such as education, income, and socioeconomic status.

Table 3-8
Cancer Outcomes: Correlational and Epidemiological Studies

Researchers and sample	Measures	Findings
Mellemgaard et al. (1994); 368 cancer cases, 396 controls; ages 20 to 79. Random sample of cancer patients with age and sex-matched controls, followed from 1989–1992.	Occupational physical activity classification, leisure physical activity, odds ratio risk of renal cell carcinoma.	(+) Women who were active in free time were at lower risk. (−) No difference in risk by occupational physical activity for either sex. No difference by age.
Levi et al. (1993); 274 cancer cases; 572 controls; female; ages 31 to 75. Endometrial cancer; convenience sample 1988–1991.	Self-rated physical activity: re housework, stairs, walking, sports, occupational. Relative risk of endometrial cancer by level of physical activity.	(+) Systematic tendency for cancer cases to report lower levels of physical activity. The association was stronger in older ages. Causal direction not clear.
Shu et al. (1993); 268 cases; 268 controls; ages 18 to 74 (avg. age = 56); Random sample of cancer patients with controls age-matched within 2 yrs; 1988–1990.	Occupational physical activity: energy expenditure, sit time; leisure physical activity: self-rated energy expenditure over 40 years.	(+) Self-rated inactive adults were at higher risk of endometrial cancer. Among working adults only, those with sedentary jobs were at higher risk.
Pukkala et al. (1993); 278 Finnish phys. ed. teachers randomly selected from possible 1,499; 278 language arts teachers from possible 8,619. All female; ages 20 to 75. Taught between 1967–1991; 202 phys. ed. (73%), 180 language arts (65%) followed up.	Occupational and leisure physical activity, diet, alcohol, tobacco. Physical activity by age. Site of cancer. Standardized incidence rates (SIR).	(−) None of the differences between SIRs for phys ed and language arts teachers was statistically significant. Phys. ed. teachers were significantly more physically active.

(Continued)

Table 3-8
(*Continued*)

Researchers and sample	Measures	Findings
Sturgeon et al. (1993); 405 cases, 297 controls, ages 20 to 74. Females with endometrial cancer. Controls randomly sampled and age-matched within 5 yrs. Followed 1987–1990. 66% sample attrition due to death, not replaced.	Self-rated physical activity in housework, stairs, walking, sports, occupational. Recent and lifetime physical activity, cancer incidence.	(+) Lifetime sedentary women may be at increased risk of endometrial cancer.
Shephard (1992); 10,224 males; 3,120 females, attending a preventive medical exam. Followed 8 years. 95% adherence.	Smoking status. Fitness levels. Cancer deaths.	(+) Inverse gradient between fitness and cancer, taking into account smoking as a factor.
Vetter et al. (1992); 87 male, 13 female cancer patients; 371 controls (random). Ages 14 to 97 yrs, median = 50. Non-colon cancer patients. 1979–1984.	Sitting Scale (motionless posture). Odds ratio linear trends of P.A. (energy expenditure) and groups (patient vs. control).	(+) Energy expenditure was the only measure to reach significance, and demonstrated increased risk for non-colon cancer.
Satariano et al. (1991); 422 breast cancer patients; 478 controls; ages 55 to 84. Random sample from 1984–1985. 3- and 12-month questionnaire. 90% response follow-up.	Physical Functional Rating included strength and range of motion measures. Odds ratio between case and control on physical function by age groups.	(+) Cancer cases had significantly lower strength and flexibility than matched controls, except oldest group (increased number of chronic diseases). No difference in physical function between three and 12 months except for the youngest group which regained function.

(*Continued*)

Table 3-8
(*Continued*)

Researchers and sample	Measures	Findings
Whitemore et al. (1990); 432 cases in China; 12,000 matched controls; 473 cases in Canada/United States, 1,192 matched controls, ages 20 to 79. From cancer clinics in China, USA, and Canada. Follow-up of 54% to 64% of subjects.	Time spent daily on physical activity: occupational physical activity; walking, taking stairs, cycling. Colorectal cancer odds ratio by 5 yr. age groups and patterns of activity.	(+) Colorectal cancer risk was elevated in men employed in sedentary occupations. In both cases, risk increased with time spent sitting. High fat intake and physical inactivity could account for 60% of colorectal cancer incidence among Chinese-American men and 40% among women.
Gerhardsson et al. (1990); Random sample (from 1968–1988) of 452 colon cancer patients; 268 rectal cancer patients; 624 controls. Ages 48 to 87. Born in Stockholm, Sweden; 50% lived independently.	Cancer incidence, year of birth, occupational and leisure time physical activity.	(+) Low physical activity levels in 1980 associated with increased risk of colon cancer for both men and women. 57% of left colon cancer risk is explained by low physical activity and dietary fat. (−) No relationship for rectal cancer.
Slattery et al. (1990); 231 randomly selected cancer cases; 391 matched controls; ages 40 to 79 yrs. Followed 3 years (71% cases, 74% controls).	Physical activity 2–3 yrs. prior; diet, occupational activity. Fitness categories were compared to occupations.	(+) Support that physical activity reduces cancer risk.

Furthermore, some of the physical activity measures were not validated, and re-call was considered a potential bias. Comparisons between studies using different instrumentation is difficult. It is essential that standardized tools be developed for assessing levels and intensities for all activities relating to active living, exercise, and physical activity. These must include appropriate activities for age-specific populations. Also, some studies have not used control groups at all, or have used controls having unrelated illnesses or disabilities.

A deeper understanding of the physiological basis for observed associations between cancer and active living is needed. This should include examination of the relationship of physical activity and the immune response. Also, more cross-cultural studies may increase our understanding since we know that there is a much higher prevalence of cancer in North America than in all the less industrialized countries. Even populations from European industrialized countries have a lower cancer risk. It may be useful to examine how cancer risks among different cultures are influenced by genetic, environmental, lifestyle, psychological, and socioeconomic factors.

DIABETES OUTCOMES

Summary

The level of evidence for the relationship between physical activity and diabetes outcomes is **indicative**. Diabetes mellitus is a metabolic disorder where the body has difficulty transporting and utilizing glucose (Durak, 1989). This can be due to the failure of the body to produce insulin (Type 1), or to a decreased sensitivity of the body to insulin (Type 2). Type 2 non-insulin-dependent diabetes mellitus (NIDDM) accounts for 90% of the diabetic population, and is most often associated with obesity (Durak, 1989; Ruderman et al., 1992). Type 2 diabetics make enough insulin, but simply have too much body mass. In contrast, Type 1 diabetics cannot produce enough insulin due to a dysfunctional pancreas, and thus are insulin-dependent (IDDM).

In turn, with blood sugar levels being consistently high, the blood becomes more viscous, and circulatory complications can become a major concern. In addition, cardiovascular disease, kidney failure, blindness, gangrene, sexual impotence, congenital abnormalities, and early mortality are common complications of this disease (Williams, 1987; Ruderman & Schneider, 1992).

Type 2 diabetes mellitus is quickly becoming a common disease, especially for overweight and sedentary individuals (Durak, 1989). The rapid increase of diabetes mellitus has been attributed to recent changes in our lifestyle (Ekoe, 1989). In Canada, for example, even with the "ParticipACTION" fitness movement beginning in the 1970s, too many Canadians today are out of shape, unfit, and over-fat. These characteristics provide an unfortunate foundation for becoming a high-risk individual for diabetes (Eck et al., 1992). Although heredity does play a small role in this disease, for the most part it can be controlled and even prevented by participating in regular physical activity (Rooney, 1993; Williams, 1987).

For Type 1 diabetes (IDDM), exercise, diet, and medication can help stabilize glucose levels. Exercise can be applied to Type 2 diabetes (NIDDM) but because obesity is often associated with NIDDM, individuals with the latter often have difficulties in moving and hence exercising. The weight and size/shape of their bodies may seriously interfere with mobility.

Although NIDDM individuals must be monitored carefully in exercise programs because of their vulnerability to pre-coronary conditions, exercise is considered to be one of the most important factors in the treatment of the diabetic patient (Staten, 1991). Maintenance of blood glucose at a more even level is one major benefit of exercise for the diabetic patient (Durak, 1989). Glucose is taken in by the cells much more readily when there are increased energy demands by the body. As well, glycogen is stored in the muscles and the liver, providing a glucose reservoir for periods of low blood sugar. Additionally, long-term training and lower blood glucose levels increase insulin sensitivity within the body (Durak, 1989). When insulin resistance is decreased, a lower dose of insulin is required for the diabetic patient. This is beneficial because it provides the individual with a wider therapeutic window in the treatment of his or her condition.

Given the effects on blood glucose and insulin sensitivity, diabetics can realize similar health benefits from exercise to those seen in the general population (Wallberg-Henriksson, 1989). Diabetics can obtain a more favorable body composition, decreased risk of heart disease, increased metabolic rate, decreased risk of osteoporosis, and enhanced feelings of well-being (Williams, 1987). However, it should be noted that most of the studies concerning exercise and diabetes have involved men and more research with women is needed to clarify unique effects by gender.

Discussion of the Evidence

A number of studies have been conducted dealing with the issue of physical activity for the aging diabetic patient. In general, most of the studies have found regular physical activity to be beneficial in the treatment of diabetes, especially Type 2. Kirwan et al. (1993) evaluated the effects of nine months of vigorous exercise training (at 80% of maximum heart rate) on the glucose-stimulated response and glucose disposal rate in 12 people age 65 with normal glucose tolerance. Artificial hyperglycemia was introduced to examine insulin action with and without exercise. At the end of the study, aerobic power had increased 23% in response to the exercise program. Insulin action was significantly improved indicating that regular exercise was effective in reducing hyperinsulemia and improving insulin action in 65-year-olds to levels typical of young adults.

Thirteen older men (61 to 82 years) were studied by Kahn et al. (1990) for the effects of exercise on insulin action, glucose tolerance, and insulin secretion. After six months of intensive exercise, maximum oxygen consumption increased 18%. An unchanged fasting glucose despite a reduced fasting insulin level suggested exercise training improved insulin sensitivity. No control group was used in their study.

Kohl et al. (1992) conducted a prospective study of 8,715 men (average age 42) and followed them for 8.2 years to determine the association of baseline cardiorespiratory fitness to all-cause mortality across various blood glucose levels. Regardless of glycemic status, fit men had lower age-adjusted all-cause death rates than their less fit counterparts. Multivariate analyses, controlling for risk factors for mortality (age, resting systolic blood pressure, serum cholesterol, body mass index, family history of heart disease, follow-up interval, smoking habit) showed a greater risk of death due to all causes for unfit compared to fit men which ranged from a relative risk of 1.38 to 1.92. Longitudinal, prospective studies are a well-respected source of scientific information. This study lends support to the theory that exercise has a preventive role for adult-onset diabetes.

Weber et al. (1983) studied 70 individuals (43 men, 27 women) between the ages of 70 and 88 to examine the effects of a diet high in complex carbohydrates, a low fat diet, and daily exercise on older adults for a 26-day period. Of the 70 adults, 13 were NIDDM-affected. Two patients were on oral hypoglycemic agents at entry, and one patient was receiving insulin injection. By the end of the study, insulin had been discontinued on one patient, and oral medication was discontinued in another. The remaining 11 participants all showed a significant improvement in glucose management. The problems with this study were that there was no control group, diet and exercise were confounded, and the number of NIDDM patients were few. Although the sample was not necessarily a good representation of the aging diabetic population, the results obtained were similar to the findings of younger adult studies which show clearly that exercise, diet, and diabetes are interrelated.

A few studies counter the evidence that older diabetics can benefit from exercise. A study of 16 males, average age 60, showed that physical training was not feasible as a treatment for older NIDDM patients (Skarfors et al., 1987). Only two participants of the eight in the training group remained for the two-year duration of the study. Of the six men who withdrew, two patients developed coronary heart disease, two suffered from metabolic disturbances, and two simply dropped out. Skarfors et al. (1987) claimed that studies on adults in an age group 10 years younger have fewer drop-outs, higher rates of improvement, and less physical ailments to complicate the research design.

This was not the only study undermined by drop-out problems. A 10-year study by Schneider et al. (1992) had problems with multiple disease conditions in its sample of diabetic patients. There were 255 diabetic patients ranging from 49 to 56 years and, of these, 174 were NIDDM patients. Again the high occurrence of health complications resulted in many participants dropping out. The perception was that exercise was complicating the disease for the diabetic older adult by increasing susceptibility to infarction, arrhythmias, and hip fractures. Another concern was the susceptibility to hypoglycemia, a risk which increases with age (Brown & Jackson, 1994).

In younger-age adults, and in some studies on older people, the benefits of active lifestyles are apparent. Rogers (1989) concluded that there is a normalization of glucose tolerance which is largely credited to regular exercise involvement. According to Rogers, exercise has an insulin-like effect on glucose transport into the muscle, whereby the muscle more readily accepts glucose across its membranes, hence lowering blood sugar levels. This effect can be seen for an extended period of time after the cessation of exercise. As well, there is a decreased resistance of the body to insulin after exercising at a submaximal level (68% VO_2max), therefore helping to stabilize blood sugar levels further (Rogers, 1989). Still to be confirmed is whether the effects of higher-intensity exercise will have a stronger effect on glucose metabolism.

Some research that has not shown decreases in blood glucose per se has shown other effects beneficial to diabetics. For example, Page et al. (1993) used a randomized control group study to determine whether impaired glucose tolerance and associated risk factors for cardiovascular disease could be improved with diet and exercise. The double-blind study lasted for six months in an outpatient environment. Participants exercised a minimum of three times each week at a sports center. The exercise program was a mixture of aerobic and anaerobic exercises: circuit training, swimming, and weight training. Dietary advice was given individually to the 37 subjects between 18 and 60 years. The placebo group showed no change in plasma glucose, cholesterol, or blood pressure. The "healthy living" group, after exclusion of four noncompliant subjects, showed no change in blood glucose levels, but a significantly decreased systolic blood pressure, and decreased plasma cholesterol. These metabolic responses were considered to decrease the risks of both diabetes and cardiovascular disease.

Although most of the evidence discussed here is from studies of NIDDM diabetics, there appear to be benefits of exercise for the IDDM adult as well. Regular physical activity has been shown to normalize peripheral insulin resistance as well as to decrease blood glucose concentrations (Wallberg-Henriksson, 1989). In addition, IDDM adults should exercise for the same health reasons as the general population with a number of cautions: diabetic exercisers must learn to make necessary adjustments in their diet according to their activity levels. IDDM patients are advised to become expert on how their bodies respond to physical activity, and accommodate their physiology accordingly.

MORTALITY OUTCOMES

Summary

The level of evidence for a link between physical inactivity and premature mortality is **indicative** for men and **suggestive** for women. Evidence that physical activity can reduce the risk of premature death from chronic diseases is growing. Consistent and positive relationships have been found between physical activity and decreased premature mortality. Moreover, an inverse gradient and dose-response relationship (up to a point) are evident. Protective effects of physical activity appear to occur to age 80 years and beyond. Moderate, low-risk physical activities appear to have greater protective effect than vigorous activity with older adults.

The studies which examined cause-specific mortality reported a stronger relationship for activity/fitness and mortality from cardiovascular disease than from cancer. This might be because of the influence of the external environment—not assessed in these studies—on cancer. More research is needed.

Most research to date has involved males; more is needed with females. However, the patterns of evidence at this point seem to be similar for women as for men, though women may gain greater benefits from moderate activity levels. More research needs to assess fitness level as well as self-reported activity, and to examine other lifestyle behaviors and health conditions. A stronger operational distinction between moderate and vigorous activity is also needed along with clarification of the nature of the relationship between activity and mortality from causes other than cardiovascular disease.

Discussion of the Evidence

This section focuses mainly on studies reported in the 1990s; which contain older subjects and have longer follow-up periods than most earlier studies. Some research reported in the 1980s which included large older adult subgroups is also discussed (Kaplan et al., 1987).

Most of the studies reviewed are prospective, and employ inclusion criteria or statistical adjustments to control for the influence of other variables that could influence mortality (e.g., age, gender, weight, smoking, family history, health status). The long follow-up periods of many of the studies reduce the possible influence of preselection on the results (e.g., Lindsted et al., 1987). If follow-up is short, it is possible that inactivity at baseline is due to the effects of illness immediately preceding death (Kaplan et al., 1987; Rakowski & Mor, 1992).

There appears to be a consistent inverse relationship between physical activity and mortality. The odds ratios or proportional hazard estimates reported in Table 3–9 suggest a dose-response relationship. That is, the more vigorous the activity (at least to a point), the lower the risk of premature death. However, several researchers have noted the rather crude estimates of exercise intensity (e.g., grouping self-reported activity levels into approximate energy expenditure categories with sometimes arbitrary cut-off points). It is possible that some of the activity classified as vigorous might be more accurately labeled as moderate.

Two of the studies reported (Bokovoy & Blair, 1994; Sandvik et al., 1993) assessed actual fitness level, rather than self-reported physical activity. As with physical activity, there was an inverse relationship between physical fitness measures and mortality. It is well accepted by exercise scientists that physical activity is the main determinant of fitness level.

The inverse gradient in the fitness-mortality relationship may be less steep for women than for men. For example, Bokovoy and Blair (1994) found that both moderately and highly fit older women had a lower all-cause mortality risk than unfit women, but the groups of fit women did not differ from each other. By contrast, older men showed more of the conventional inverse gradient pattern, with a large risk difference between highly fit and unfit men, and a moderate difference (approaching significance) between moderately and highly fit men. A similar pattern was evident for cardiovascular disease mortality.

Why the gradient appears less steep for women is unclear. Perhaps there is a wider range of fitness levels among men, given that leisure time sports and physical activities have until recently been more common among males. Or is there a larger difference in fitness between moderately and highly fit men than between moderately and highly fit women? Another explanation is that unfit women may be less fit than unfit men, so females may reap greater benefits of achieving a moderate level of fitness.

There appear to be no gender differences between self-reported physical activity and all-cause mortality (Rehm et al., 1993; Simonsick et al., 1993), or mortality from cardiovascular disease or cancer (Rehm et al., 1993). However, the type of activity that is predictive may differ between women and men. Rakowski and Mor (1992) found that for men, estimated activity compared to peers and to what men believe is "enough exercise" were most predictive of mortality. For women, walking a mile at least once per week was most predictive. Those authors have suggested that in making negative comparisons with peers or a perceived ideal, men may be expressing an accurate perception of being unfit and therefore at higher risk. Rakowski and Mor have suggested that reported walking may have

Table 3-9
Mortality Outcomes: Correlational and Epidemiological Studies

Researchers and sample	Measures	Findings
Bokovoy and Blair (1994); 2,054 females, 6,878 males; ages 50 and over. Adults receiving medical exams at Cooper Aerobics Clinic, Dallas, Texas for 19 yrs; avg follow-up, 8 yrs. 77 (3.4%) women and 513 (7.5%) men died.	Fitness levels: high (most fit 40%); moderate (next 40%); low (least fit 20%); assessed by treadmill max test. Deaths/ 10,000 person yrs. of follow-up; adjusted by age; from gov't mortality statistics.	(+) High fit men and women had significantly lower all-cause mortality rates. All cause: low fit men, Relative Risk (RR) = 3.32 vs. high fit men; low fit women, RR = 2.37 vs. moderately fit women. CVD: low fit men, RR = 5.23 vs. fit men; low fit women, RR = 2.98 vs. high fit women. Relationship held across all 5-year age groups regardless of health status for men (sample too small to evaluate for women).
Paffenbarger et al. (1993); 10,269 males, ages 45 to 84 in 1977 at time of final lifestyle survey (avg. age 57.5 ± 8.8). Harvard alumni (1916–1950), no diagnosed chronic diseases (e.g., CHD, cancer), followed until age 85. 2 groups: < 2000 kcal/week = sedentary, > 2000 kcal/week = active. Followed 23 yrs, plus archival records from student days; last 9 years of interest in this study; 68% lifestyle survey return rate in 1962/1966; 76% for 1977 follow-up; 476 (4.6%) deaths from 1977–1985.	Blocks walked, stairs climbed daily; type, frequency, duration of sports (hrs/week). Sedentary vs. active groups. Controlled for age, smoking, alcohol, close relationships. Diet not assessed. All-cause and CHD mortality, 1977–1985; (from Harvard Alumni Office and gov't stats); longevity estimate (years of life added).	(+) Sedentary men had 25% higher all-cause death risk and 36% higher CHD death risk. If climbed < 20 flights of stairs/week: 23% higher all-cause risk, 56% higher CHD risk. If no moderately vigorous sports: 44% higher all-cause risk, 51% higher CHD risk. Men who increased to > 2000 kcal/week energy expenditure from 1962–1966 to 1977: 15% lower all-cause risk and 17% lower CHD risk. If started moderately vigorous sport: 23% less all-cause risk, 41% lower CHD risk. Estimated .72 year of life added if start moderately vigorous sport; 2.49 years added if start sport and also quit smoking.

(Continued)

Table 3-9
(Continued)

Researchers and sample	Measures	Findings
Rehm et al. (1993); 489 females, 419 males, ages 30 to 69 in 1975–1977 (379 age 60 and over; 328 age 45 to 59). German, random rural community sample. Followed 13 yrs. 85% of 1975–1977 sample completed the study.	Self-reported physical activity during physician interviews (none, occasional, regular). Control for age, disease, alcohol, smoking, close relationships. Mortality between 1975–1977 and 1988–1990; from gov't stats.	(+) Mortality risk lowest for regular physical activity (RR = .32 women, .57 men); some protective effect for occasional activity (RR = .50 women, .76 men). Activity most protective for CHD and cancer (but small subsamples for latter). Women who were inactive **and** heavy drinkers at very high risk. (RR = 21.63).
Sandvik et al. (1993); 1960 males, ages 40 to 59 between 1972–1975 (avg. age 50). Employees of 5 Norwegian companies, both white and blue collar, no diagnosed diseases at start of the study. 15.9 yrs. avg. follow-up .6% of workers participated. 271 (13.8%) died by 1989.	Fitness level assessed by bicycle ergometer VO_2 max test; sample divided into fitness quartiles (Q1 = low fitness). Study adjusted for age, smoking, cholesterol, blood pressure, BMI, vital capacity, resting heart rate, physical activity behavior (active vs. not active). Mortality between 1972–1975 and 1989 from gov't stats.	(+) For all-cause mortality: High fit men (Q4) had lower risk than men in other three quartiles (RR = .54 vs. Q1, .59 vs. Q2, .53 vs. Q3). For CHD mortality: Q4 and Q3 lower risk vs. Q1 (RR = .41 and .45). Q4 marginally signif. ($p = .06$) lower risk vs. Q3 (RR = .50).
Kaplan et al. (1987); 4,174 adults, no gender data. At least age 38 in 1965; (890 ages 65 to 70; 564 age 70+). Residents of Alameda, California; racial mix, various income levels. Followed 17 yrs. 1,219 (29%) died by 1982.	Self-reported frequency of leisure time physical activity; survey questionnaire controlled for six other health behaviors: smoking, relative weight, alcohol, sleep, breakfast, snacking. Mortality (all cause); gov't stats (California and other states).	(+) For those over 60 yrs of age: low activity associated with increased mortality risk vs. high activity (RR = 1.38). No difference between 60–69 and 70+. Similar results for age 50–59 (RR = 1.27).

(Continued)

Table 3-9
(*Continued*)

Researchers and sample	Measures	Findings
Simonsick et al. (1993); 2,913 females, 2,264 males, 65 and over in 1982. Prospective study. East Boston, two Iowa counties (whole community sampled), New Haven, Connecticut (random sample); multi-race sample. Excluded those with functional disabilities. 3-, 6-year follow-ups (78% to 91% of subjects). 1,186 (22.9%) died.	Self-reported physical activity in leisure time or home maintenance; 16% to 26% classified as high active (vigorous activity or sport); 46% to 57% as moderately active, 26% to 32% as inactive. Controlled for self-rated health status, education, smoking, depression, chronic conditions. Mortality from annual follow-up household interviews and obituaries.	(+) 3-yr. follow-up: Highly active people had lower mortality risk than inactive people (RR significant for Iowa only, at .45); no difference between moderate and inactive. 6-yr. follow-up: RR for highly active vs. inactive significant for Iowa and New Haven (.59 and .66); no difference moderate active vs. inactive; similar for women and men.
Koiso and Ohsawa (1992); 3,113 males; avg. age of death 65. Retrospective, records of former university students, years 1872–1981. Both university major and death records retrospective.	Compared phys. ed. with humanities and science majors; no measure of physical activity either when in school or over life span. Mortality (all causes); measured both as age at death and by Cutler, Ederer cumulative survival rates.	(−) This study did not examine actual physical activity. Phys. ed. majors lived 5 to 8 years less than humanities and science majors. (Similar results when war deaths were included vs. excluded).

(*Continued*)

Table 3-9
(Continued)

Researchers and sample	Measures	Findings
Rakowski and Mor (1992); U.S. national sample 3,679 females, 2,222 males; age 70 and over (2,588 ages 70 to 74; 1,859 age 75 to 79; 945 ages 80 to 85; 509 age 85+). Under-representation of people who were older, less formal education, non-Caucasian, experiencing health problems. Followed 4 years, 13% (879) of original 6,780 not traced for 1988; 1,098 (18.6%) died.	1984 self-assessment of activity relative to peers; getting enough exercise; frequency of 1-mile walks during week; having a regular exercise schedule. Adjusted for daily functioning, age, gender, social networks. Mortality during 1984–1988 from follow-up survey and gov't records.	(+) All 4 physical activity measures predicted mortality. Females: highest age-adjusted odds ratio was for women who walked a mile never or once per week (RR = 2.5). Males: Being less active than peers and not getting enough exercise were most predictive (RR = 1.37 and 1.77). Subjects with limitations in daily functioning: walking a mile never or once per week most predictive of mortality (RR = 2.30).
Sarna et al. (1992); 2,613 male athletes (303 endurance, 909 power, 1,185 team sports); 1,712 in reference group. Athletes: mean age 60 to 73 in 1989 (depending on sport); Finnish athletes from Olympics or other international games between 1920–1965. Nonathletic referents: mean age 67; men fit for compulsory military service at age 20. Deaths among athletes ranges from 17.9% to 51.9% among athletes in various sports; 41.8% for referents.	Subjects classified in 1978–1979; questionnaire on background characteristics and lifestyle behavior in 1985; vital status examined in 1989. Adjustments for occupational and marital status, age of entry into cohort. Mortality from records of vital statistics from gov't (military service deaths excluded).	(+) Life expectancy (LE) estimates were highest for endurance athletes (LE = 75.6); next highest for team athletes (LE = 73.9), power athletes (LE = 71.5), then the reference group (LE=69.9). Endurance athletes had lower all-cause mortality risk than other groups (RR = .59). Endurance and team athletes had lower CHD death risk (RR = .49 and .61); endurance and power athletes had lower cancer risk (RR = .36 and .55). Power athletes had high risk from external causes of death vs. other groups (RR = 2.0). More athletes than referents reported doing regular physical activity in 1985.

(Continued)

Table 3-9
(*Continued*)

Researchers and sample	Measures	Findings
Lindsted et al. (1991); 9,484 males, avg. age: 49.9 for highly active; 54.7 for moderately active; 51.6 for inactive. Prospective study; seventh day adventists, (California) followed from 1960 lifestyle survey through to 1985. 26 years, 15 yr avg follow-up time; 4,000 (42%) died during follow-up.	Self-reported exercise at work or play, on 1960 lifestyle survey (1,609 highly active; 5,803 moderately active; 2,072 inactive. Controlled for education, race, marital status, smoking, nutrition, BMI, disease. All cause and disease-specific mortality from gov't records; poisonings, accidents, congenital causes excluded; examined trends across 10-yr. age intervals.	(+) All-cause mortality: both moderate and high active groups had fewer deaths than inactive; protective effect (RR significant < 1) beyond 80 yrs for moderate activity, but lost significance at age 70 for high activity. Cardiovascular diseases: significant protective effect of moderate activity up to age 80, but not high activity (trend to age 70). Cancer: no significant effects, but trend for moderate activity up to 70 years. Crossover of risk (when RR > 1, occurred at a younger age for high active group for all causes of death.

(*Continued*)

Table 3-9
(Continued)

Researchers and sample	Measures	Findings
Morris et al. (1990); 9,376 males; lifestyle questionnaire for random sample of 25% (2,344 males). Ages 45 to 64; (4,552 age 45 to 54; 4,824 age 55 to 64). Executives in British civil service; middle class; sedentary or physically light office work. Those with CHD history excluded. 9.3 years avg. follow-up; 289 (3%) died.	Four levels of self-reported physical activity intensity. Level 1 = vigorous sports such as walking, cycling at least 2 times/week (216 males); level 2 = vigorous activity less than twice but more than once/week, or more frequent but less intense activity (424 males); level 3 = occasional sports (1 to 3 times/mo), or short brisk walks (519 males); 4 = no vigorous activity (1,185 males). Study controlled for smoking, BMI, age, family history, stature, subclinical CVD. Examined deaths due to coronary heart disease from gov't stats.	(+) Group 1 (most vigorous) demonstrated lower mortality risk vs. other 3 groups for ages 45 to 54 (RR% = 25); Groups 1 and 2 had lower risk vs. other 2 groups for ages 55 to 64 (RR% = 53 and 59).
Quinn et al. (1990); 348 males (185 athletes; 163 non-athletes. Avg. age 69 in 1976. Prospective study of males who completed the 1976 and 1984 surveys of the Minnesota State University longitudinal study, or who had completed the 1976 survey but had died by 1984 (study started in 1952). Follow-up was 8 years for the present analyses with older adults. 11.5% deaths in youngest cohort (1915–1920), 58.2% in oldest (1885–1999) between 1952–1984.	Self-reported lifestyle behavior including physical activity (Minnesota Leisure Time Physical Activity Ques.). Subjects grouped by caloric expenditure per week; no adjustments for other variables in mortality analysis due to small sample size. Mortality rates examined.	(−) This was one of the few studies that did not show an inverse physical activity-mortality relationship. Unadjusted death rates were much higher in lower energy expenditure groups. However, when birth year and cardiovascular disease were considered, neither energy expenditure or athletic status predicted mortality in logistic regression analysis.

been predictive for women but not men because men were closer to the age of average life expectancy for their gender. All subjects in that study were over 70.

There may be differential benefits of moderate versus vigorous physical activity for sedentary compared to more active older adults, with the sedentary achieving more health gains from moderate activity. Morris et al. (1990) suggested that because oxygen transport mechanisms and work capacity decline with age, less intense exercise may still have significant cardiorespiratory training effects for older adults. They found that for their older cohort (55 to 64), lower mortality rates were associated with both vigorous and moderate activity, whereas in the younger cohort (45 to 54), only the vigorous activity subgroup had a lower death rate. Morris et al. stressed the importance of regular, rhythmic, large muscle movements, finding that vigorous (e.g., digging) or moderate (e.g., lawn mowing) recreational activity did not predict mortality. They suggested that such vigorous activities were done too sporadically to be beneficial.

Physical activity has been shown to exert a protective effect against premature mortality beyond age 80 (Lindsted et al., 1991; Bokovoy & Blair, 1994). Furthermore, Paffenbarger et al. (1993) found that men who took up physical activity late in life gained the same benefits as their classmates who were active throughout their lifetimes.

An important issue in the physical activity-mortality relationship is the age at crossover of risk, or the point at which physical activity no longer improves mortality risk (relative risk crosses 1.00). Lindsted et al. (1991) found that this age was higher for moderate than for vigorous activity. They have suggested that the age at crossover of risk is consistent with the hypothesis that frail individuals may postpone mortality through activity, then be at increased mortality risk as they approach the end of the human life span. However, the authors also suggested that unmeasured risk factors, different genetic susceptibilities among groups, or changes in physical activity and other risk factors over time could explain age at crossover of risk. More research is needed to determine what age groups benefit most from which levels of physical activity, and when diminishing returns begin to occur.

One weakness in the physical activity-mortality studies is the reliance by many of them on self-report. People may find it difficult to recall or estimate their physical activity behaviors accurately. Positive response bias could also be an issue, given the awareness of physical activity as a desirable behavior. However, such bias would actually make a relationship between low activity and high mortality more difficult to find. It is important to note that

(a) the consistency of the relationship between self-reported physical activity and mortality, despite the many different types of self-report questions used, and

(b) the consistency of findings among studies which use self-reported activity compared with physiological fitness testing. Both suggest a relationship that is real and not an artifact of biases or a particular type of measurement.

Many of the studies discussed used convenience samples of university alumni, employees of large organizations, or elite athletes. In the above populations, men have been more available for research, thus greatly outnumbering women, especially in the older age groups. It is essential that more women be studied and that results based on male-only samples not be generalized to women. Also, samples have been predominantly Caucasian and middle-income (or higher). Although some studies have included other races and socioeconomic groups, sample sizes were inadequate for subgroup analyses.

Furthermore, most studies did not assess diet or control for related risk factors such as blood pressure or cholesterol levels, perhaps because of the large number of studies relying on self-report measures. Because lifestyle behaviors tend to cluster (Schoenborn, 1993), it is possible that some of the benefits credited to physical activity might actually related to other behavior changes.

Physical activity appears to offer protection for premature mortality even in the presence of other factors. For example, Blair (1993) found that low-fit women and men had higher mortality rates than their moderately and highly active peers at all levels of body mass index (BMI), suggesting that physical activity can protect even overweight people from premature mortality. Brill et al. (1992) found that a higher all-cause death rate in unfit men was not influenced by anxiety or depression, suggesting that those mental health factors do not limit physical activity's benefits for mortality. Rakowski and Mor (1992) found that adults over age 70 who had limitations in activities of daily living were at lower mortality risk if they walked a mile at least once per week. Rehm et al. (1993) found that women who were heavy drinkers *and* inactive were at higher risk than were women who drank heavily and were active. More research is needed on how health conditions and other lifestyle behaviors interact with physical activity and fitness to influence mortality.

SUDDEN DEATH OUTCOMES

Summary

The available evidence is at an **acceptable** level for the relationship between physical activity and sudden death in older adults. This means that the risks of sudden death during or subsequent to physical activity are known to be remote and fall in the range of one fatality per 500,000 to one million activity hours. Sudden death in older adults usually occurs within accustomed levels of physical activity, and is predominantly associated with coronary artery disease. Most victims are male. However, sudden deaths caused by physical activity, as a consequence of advanced and undetected heart disease, are rare.

Even serious complications in exercise programs for known heart-diseased patients are infrequent. Van Camp and Peterson (1986) observed one fatality per 750,000 patient-hours of supervised exercise and nine cardiac arrests per million patient-hours of exercise. These mortality rates are no different than would be expected in nonexercising patients of similar age. Siskovick (1990) reached similar conclusions in reviewing 20 years of large epidemiological studies.

In fact, rather than increasing risk, habitual and vigorous forms of physical activity can reduce the risk of coronary events leading to sudden death during activity. Although risk of sudden death is elevated during periods of heavy exertion, the relative risks involved in a sedentary lifestyle are even higher. Risks of coronary heart disease are increased by obesity, age, and hypertension. Also, diabetics have been shown to be at greater risk of myocardial infarction than non-diabetics. Regular, progressive, and moderate forms of physical activity are a counterbalance to these risk factors, rather than a liability.

Discussion of the Evidence

Sudden death during or after exercise appears to be primarily a male phenomenon (Ragosta et al., 1984). Sudden death as an outcome of physical activity has been examined more in younger men (often in military settings) than in older women and men. Young men with undetected heart problems may be at higher risk because of their involvement in high-exertion activities. It is not clear whether older age or sedentary lifestyle or a combination of both leads to increased risk of asymptomatic CHD leading to sudden death. More research with older men and women is needed.

There is no medical evidence that physical activity (even more vigorous forms) is harmful to a healthy cardiovascular system. On the contrary, regular physical activity is thought to provide older adults with early warning of symptoms related to disease or deficiency in the cardiovascular system (Gottlieb & Gerstenblith, 1988). The evidence from supervised cardiac rehabilitation programs among middle-age and older adults strongly supports regular vigorous physical activity as a protective influence to reduce the risks of sudden death through myocardial infarction in daily living (Van Camp & Petersen, 1986). However an individual with structural cardiovascular disease, even if asymptomatic, is at an increased risk for sudden death during vigorous forms of physical activity. Therefore supervised and graded exercise for these individuals is needed (Van Camp, 1988).

More recently, Whittington and Banerjee (1994), over a four-year period, examined all sport-related deaths that occurred within six hours of participation. Out of a British population of 1,130,000, only 52 deaths occurred. The age range was 8 to 84, but few deaths occurred in young people. In the younger subjects, death was caused by undetected congenital heart problems. Among adults, bowling and golf were the most common activities leading to sudden death. In all cases, the people were performing within accustomed levels of physical activity, but coronary artery disease was responsible in 43 of the 52 cases. Common to these sudden death events while exercising was the fact that the fatalities were asymptomatic. The researchers concluded that sudden death events are almost always related to some form of coronary artery disease. They also pointed out that currently there is no single effective prevention, and that most heart-related deaths occur in everyday activities rather than during formal exercise.

A larger study which examined relative risks of myocardial infarction by level and intensity of physical exertion reported findings consistent with the previous epidemiological results. Using a case-control design, Mittleman et al. (1993) studied 836 males and 392 females who had had a myocardial infarction, along with 218 controls, for three years (age range 22 to 92). They found that sedentary, rather than active, individuals had a much higher relative risk of myocardial infarction than those who were involved in heavy physical exertion (6+ METs), five or more times a week. Other findings of interest included:

(a) diabetics had a higher relative risk than non-diabetics;
(b) relative risk was not affected by sex, obesity, or hypertensiveness; and
(c) those in the 70+ age group were at a higher relative risk, but this was attributable to less regular exercise patterns in this group.

The incidence of sudden death during physical activity is relatively low in comparison to other mortality event statistics. Current screening methods such as pre-activity medical exams (including stress tests) may not always find underlying problems; asymtomatic problems may result in sudden death when triggered by physical exertion.

As previously mentioned, most incidences of activity-related sudden death are among men. More men than women are active in sport and exercise at every life stage, and men tend to choose more vigorous activities. However, more women have fatal outcomes of first heart attacks. Research is needed to clarify whether the same rates of sudden death occur when women are equally active, and how the circumstances surrounding sudden death among women and men may differ.

The other area which has not been adequately explored is whether or not age is associated with increased risk of activity-related sudden death. It would be useful to examine if the aging process itself puts one at risk, or whether age as a risk factor is complicated by altered lifestyle patterns associated with aging. These issues are important to address soon because more adults are entering their middle years and contemplating the personal risks involved in physical activity.

Chapter 4

Psychosocial Outcomes

ANXIETY OUTCOMES

Summary

Evidence for a link between exercise and anxiety reduction is **inconclusive**. Anxiety arises when an individual perceives a high degree of uncertainty and lack of control over demands, resources, behavioral consequences and their meaning, and bodily reactions. Negative cognitive appraisal of uncertainty and lack of control is accompanied by increased physiological arousal as well as feelings of worry, self-doubt, and apprehension. Moderate to high levels of arousal negatively affect task performance, through effects on perception, retention, and decision making (Landers & Petruzello, 1994).

Cross-sectional and correlational studies are relatively consistent in showing physically fit people experience less anxiety than unfit people. Individuals who are initially unfit or high-anxious achieve the greatest reductions in anxiety from an exercise program. While evidence is inconclusive as to the anxiety-reducing effect of exercise on healthy populations, ill and institutionalized patients seem to benefit. Also, while there is evidence of the benefits of activity for reducing anxiety among populations, these results are not directly applicable to the elderly. Correlational studies show a stronger link than intervention studies. More research is needed into what frequency, duration, and intensity of exercise is needed to obtain anxiety reduction, and what physiological (e.g., neurochemical) and psychological (e.g., distraction) mechanisms mediate between increased exercise and reduced anxiety.

Discussion of the Evidence

Anxiety is commonly understood to be of two types–state and trait anxiety. Trait anxiety is believed to be a relatively stable personality trait concerning one's predisposition to anxiety; it is somewhat susceptible to alteration. In contrast, state anxiety is a transient situation of worry associated with a specific event or circumstance. Research has attempted mainly to detect changes in trait anxiety. The studies discussed in this section deal with trait anxiety unless otherwise indicated.

Little research has been done on state anxiety, though studies with younger subjects has shown that state anxiety was reduced with both chronic and acute bouts of exercise (Petruzzello et al., 1991; Roth, 1989). Also, continuous (aerobic) rather than intermittent (anaerobic) movements appear to be more strongly associated with reductions in anxiety (Landers & Petruzzello, 1994).

Although some studies support reduced anxiety accompanying exercise intervention (King et al., 1993; Richardson & Rosenberg, 1989; Minor et al., 1989), others have found no effect (Blumenthal et al., 1991; Emery & Gatz, 1990). Emery and Blumenthal (1991) offered an excellent review of the inconsistent pattern of findings among older adults.

King et al. (1993) investigated the effects of differing intensities of exercise on anxiety levels in older adults. The sample ($N = 357$) was separated into four intervention groups varying by exercise intensity: control, high-intensity–group program, high-intensity–home program, and low-intensity–home program. After 12 months, exercisers reported significantly lower anxiety scores than controls. Exercise intensity was not related to anxiety outcomes.

Blumenthal et al. (1989, 1991), in reporting on the 4- and 14-month results of the Duke Aging and Exercise Study, failed to find any significant changes in anxiety scores as a result of exercise participation. An earlier study (Blumenthal et al., 1982) also failed to find any significant changes in anxiety among elderly participants in an exercise program. Emery & Gatz (1990) found similar results.

Research on institutionalized patients has produced controversial findings. Gayle et al. (1988) found that trait, but not state, anxiety was consistently reduced as a function of participation in an exercise program with COPD patients. Because the anxiety measures were administered up to a week after the last exercise session (3 exercise periods), events other than exercise could have influenced anxiety levels.

In contrast, Emery (1994) found significant reductions in both anxiety and depression a 30-day exercise program with 64 COPD patients (mean age 67.4 years). In work with rheumatoid arthritic and osteoarthritic patients, Minor et al. (1989) found significant declines in anxiety for those subjects in an exercise program.

Table 4-1

Anxiety Outcomes: Intervention and Comparison Studies

Researchers and sample	Design, treatment, and measures	Findings
Emery (1994); 64 older adults (29 F, 35M), ages 53 to 82. Two age groups: younger, avg. age = 67.4; older, avg. age = 73.1. Older out-patient convenience sample; pulmonary rehab program at Duke University's Center for Living (55% male). No control group.	Small group program for 30 days; 4 hours/ session: respiratory therapy plus warm-up floor exercises, 45 min aerobic exercise and Nautilus strength training; 5 days/week; no intensity level reported. 95% adherence. Anxiety measured by the Psychological General Well-Being Index (Dupuy, 1974); 3 measures of aerobic fitness: forced vital capacity, VO_2max using cycle ergometry and timed 12 minute walk for distance.	(+) Significant declines in symptom check list anxiety for both age groups. Significant improvement in all 3 aerobic measures of fitness.
King et al. (1993); 357 older adults (160 F, 197 M). Avg. age 57 (range 50 to 65). Participants recruited from a random-digit-dial telephone survey, Sunnyvale, CA. Absence of cardio-vascular disease, no regular exercise program.	Four groups: (1) High-intensity group = based exercise, at local senior center, 60 min 3 times/wk; 12 months; 73% to 88% max HR; (2) high-intensity home-based exercise, 60 min 3 times/wk, 12 months; 73% to 88% max HR; (3) low-intensity home exercise, 30 min 5 times/wk, 12 months; 60% to 73% max HR; (4) controls, not to change habits for 12 months. Measure: Taylor Manifest Anxiety Scale (TAMS).	(+) Significantly lower anxiety scores for all exercise subjects. Significantly lower perceived anxiety scores for all exercise participants.

(Continued)

Table 4-1
(*Continued*)

Researchers and sample	Design, treatment, and measures	Findings
Gitlin et al. (1992); 267 older adults, 64% women, 36% men. Avg. age = 69 (range 60 to 89). Community residents recruited through senior centers, public announcements. All relatively healthy.	Randomized into 2 groups: bicycle exercise group; attention control group. Bicycle group: 40 min, 3 times/week for 4 months, at 70% max HR. Attention control group: met in small groups once/week, seminars on "positive lifestyles." Measure: State-Trait Anxiety Index (STAI).	(−) No significant effect on anxiety.
Gronningsaeter et al. (1992); 76 older adults ages 25 to 67. Inactive employees of an insurance company.	Randomly assigned to three groups: Physical activity intevention: 55 min, 3 sessions/ week, for ten weeks at 70% to 80% of max HR. Stress training: same frequency as exercise, educational strategies. Control group. 56% still active at 6 months of follow-up; 91% examined again at 9 months. Measure: State-Trait Anxiety Scale.	(−) No significant change in anxiety for any of the groups.
Blumenthal et al. (1991); 101 older adults ages 60 to 83. Healthy sedentary volunteers recruited through news media. 50 men; 51 women.	Conditional random assignment to 3 groups: Aerobic: 3 times/week, 30 min; yoga: 60 min, 2 times/week; control group. After 4 months wait-list subjects did aerobic exercise for remaining 10 months of study. 97 completed the 16 weeks of the study (97%); 8-month compliance was 80%. Measure: State-Trait Anxiety Inventory (STAI).	(−) No significant changes in anxiety scores; 10 to 15% improvement in peak VO_2 after 4 months; subjects comprised very healthy and motivated elderly for whom exercise benefits would not be likely to improve scores.

(*Continued*)

Table 4-1

(*Continued*)

Researchers and sample	Design, treatment, and measures	Findings
Emery and Blumenthal (1991); 64 older adults (29 F, 35 M) ages 53 to 82. Subjects recruited from an outpatient pulmonary rehab program at Duke. All have chronic obstructive pulmonary disease (COPD) > 50 years; symptoms for more than 6 months; ratio of forced expiratory vol. in 1 sec to forced vital capacity (FEV/FVC) < .70.	Participants in small groups of 5 to 8 for 30 days. Exercise: met 5 days/weeks, 4 hours/day. Sessions have sequence of respiratory therapy, warm-up, 45 min aerobic exercise. Subjects also strength trained daily and swam twice per week. Measures: Hopkins Symptom checklist (SCL-90-R). Both anxiety and depression measures. Psychological General Well-Being Scale (PGWB), both anxiety and depression measures.	(−) No differences among groups. All subjects reported less anxiety and depression. Older-old subjects reported less distress than younger subjects at both times of measurement.
Emery and Gatz (1990); 48 older adults (40 F, 8 M), avg. age = 73 (range 61 to 86). Sedentary, ethnically diverse, volunteers. 80% no education beyond high school, predominately low- and middle-income.	Control group. Randomized to one of three groups: Aerobic: 3 times/week for 12 weeks, reaching 70% max HR. Social: met 3 times/ week for 12 weeks for nonphysical activity. 19% attrition; 39 of 48 subjects completed 12 week program. Measure: CES-Scale Anxiety.	(−) No change in anxiety over 12 weeks; no significant change in blood pressure or resting heart rate; intensity of exercise is suspect.

(*Continued*)

Table 4-1
(*Continued*)

Researchers and sample	Design, treatment, and measures	Findings
Minor et al. (1989); 120 older adults. Subjects had either rheumatoid arthritis (RA), avg. age = 54 yrs; or osteoarthritis (OA), avg. age = 63 yrs. Recruited from clinics.	Subjects assigned to one of three groups: Aerobic walking; aerobic aquatics, range of motion (ROM), control group. All subjects met for 1 hour, 3 times/week, for 12 weeks. Walking and aquatic groups exercised at 60% to 80% of max HR. Five dropouts. Measures: Arthritis Impact Measurement Scale (AIMS) - Anxiety Subscales of AIMS.	(+) Significant changes for anxiety reduction for exercise groups over control groups. Aerobic and fitness measures showed significant improvement; depression also was significantly reduced.
Mittleman et al. (1989); 22 older adults (6 F, 22 M), ages 62 to 77. Healthy seniors who cycled across Canada (7700 km).	Cycling across Canada for over 100 days. Everyone cycled 6 out of every 7 days, averaging approx. 90 km/7-hour day. 11 dropouts. Measure: Spielberger State-Trait Inventory	(−) No significant change in anxiety among the already high-fit sample over the four measurement times. No sex differences in anxiety.
Richardson and Rosenberg (1989); 30 older adults ages 20 to 63. Two age groups: > 40 (avg. age = 49.1); < 40 (avg. age = 29.4). Sedentary female volunteers, healthy but not active.	All subjects participated in a 7-week walk-jog program then discontinued for 7 weeks. Purpose was to study the effects of training and detraining. All subjects did same protocol: exercise 3 times/week for 7 weeks, beginning at 60% of max capacity and progressing to 75% max. All subjects detrained for seven weeks. Measures: Comparative State Anxiety Inventory (CSAI-2) (Martens et al., 1981); 3 subscales: AS-State anxiety somatic, ASC-State anxiety self-confidence, AC-State anxiety cognitive scales.	(+) Both age groups significantly lower anxiety by end of study (AS). Older group had greater ASC at start and end of study. At end of conditioning program, no significant difference, but under 40-yr.-old adults declined at conditioning, while over 40 increased continually. No significant changes in AC. Significant changes in max HR, resting systolic BP, max treadmill time.

(*Continued*)

Table 4-1
(*Continued*)

Researchers and sample	Design, treatment, and measures	Findings
Gayle et al. (1988); 15 older adults (6 F, 9 M) ages 47 to 71. (COPD) patients.	Randomized into 2 groups: experimental ($n = 9$) and control ($n = 6$). Experimental: 2 consecutive exercise periods, 50 min 3 times/week for 14 wks., with pre/post and halfway testing. Control was the same except they did not participate in initial 14-week exercise program. Measure: Spielberg State-Trait Anxiety Inventory (STAI).	(+) Mean trait anxiety was consistently reduced as a function of exercise participation. State anxiety was below the norms.
Segebartt et al. (1988); 25 older adults aged 70 years and over. Recruited from an independent living center; Caucasian; no chronic disease or cancer, mood-altering drugs.	13 active subjects, avg. age = 80.9; 12 inactive subjects; avg. age = 81.8. Self-reported exercise. Active criteria: average 123 min/week for last 30 years. Inactive reported approx. 69 years of inactivity. Profile of Mood States (POMS).	(−) Small samples to compare. There was no difference in anxiety score between the active and inactive groups.
Shephard et al. (1987); 31 older adults (17 F, 14 M). Avg. age = 61 (range 45 to 75). Volunteers from university community.	Exercise consisted of 1 group session and 4 home sessions/week. Exercise lasted 1 hour for 20 weeks, achieving 60% of aerobic power. Adherence was 52% to complete schedule. Measure: Spielberger State-Trait Anxiety Index.	(−) Exercise produced no significant effect on anxiety scores.

(*Continued*)

Table 4-1
(Continued)

Researchers and sample	Design, treatment, and measures	Findings
Stacey et al. (1985); 66 older adults over 50. 37 active members of a fitness club, 29 new members; all volunteers.	Study divided into 2 groups: currently active and newly active. Aerobic training for a 6-month period. Exercise (1 session/wk) consisted of 30 min of stretching and aerobics, and 30 min of self-monitored swim. 16 dropouts. Measure: State-trait Anxiety Inventory (STAI).	(−) Anxiety levels were not affected throughout study. (Study also failed to obtain improvements in areobic power). Youngest, least happy, and most anxious most likely to drop out of exercise program.
Perri and Templar (1984–1985); 42 older adults (28 F, 14 M). Avg. age = 65 (range 60 to 79). Volunteers.	Control group maintained current lifestyle. Exercise consisted of walking-jogging. Exercise: 30 min aerobic (40% to 50% of max effort), 3 times/wk for 14 weeks. 17 dropouts. Measure: Zuckerman Anxiety Scale.	(+) Significant improvements in anxiety scores by exercise group.

Evidence from cross-sectional and correlational data provides stronger support for an association than has been shown in intervention studies. Frequent exercise and higher levels of fitness among elderly populations have been found to be associated with lower levels of anxiety in older populations (Stephens, 1988; Krause et al., 1993). Table 4-1 presents intervention and comparison studies; Table 4-2, correlational and epidemiological studies.

DEPRESSION OUTCOMES

Summary

Evidence of a relationship among depression, exercise, and aging is **weak**. Intervention studies have failed to support the hypothesis that exercise reduces depression for the aged, while cross-sectional research indicates some association between these variables. There is some evidence for an association between

Table 4-2
Anxiety Outcomes: Correlational and Epidemiological Studies

Researchers and sample	Measures	Findings
Stephens (1988); $N > 53,000$, all ages, 4 surveys used: National Health and Nutrition Exam Survey; Canada Health Survey; National Survey of Personal Health Practices and Consequences; Canada Fitness Survey.	Centre for Epidemiological Studies - Depression. Bradburn Affect Balance Scale. Health Opinion Survey.	(+) Level of physical activity was shown to be positively associated with lower levels of anxiety; association especially strong for women and people over 40 years of age.

reductions in depression and exercise participation among mildly to moderately depressed individuals. Recent research, however, has seriously challenged the once accepted belief that exercise has a significant effect in reducing depression when the population studied is not clinically depressed. Also, depression reductions do not seem to be associated with exercise intensity. Social participation, not high-intensity exercise, is primarily cited as prerequisite to reductions in depression. Studies which control for the social contribution of supervised exercise programming may clarify the actual contribution of physical activity to mood enhancement.

Inherent in the research, however, are methodological problems such as small samples, lack of randomized controls, and ineffective exercise protocols. Much of the research into depression and aging has either been with institutionalized populations exhibiting high levels of depression, or on voluntary populations who largely exhibit low levels of depression in their pre-test scores. Most research samples have self-selected. While initial research indicated a positive relationship, more recent studies using more rigorous methodologies have found predominantly no association.

Discussion of the Evidence

Table 4-3 presents intervention and comparison studies regarding the effects of exercise on depression. Table 4-4 presents correlational and epidemiological studies.

Table 4-3
Depression Outcomes: Intervention and Comparison Studies

Researchers and sample	Design, treatment, and measures	Findings
King et al. (1993); 357 older adults (160 F, 197 M); avg. age = 57 (range 50 to 65). Subjects recruited from a random-digit-dial telephone survey, Sunnyvale, CA. Absence of cardiovascular disease, not regularly exercising.	12-month study. 4 groups: High-intensity–group-based exercise; at local senior center, 60 min, 3 times/week, 73% to 88% max HR. High-intensity–home-based exercise; at home, 60 min, 3 times/week, 73% to 88% max HR; Low-intensity–home exercise; at home, 30 min, 5 times/week, 60% to 73% max HR; Control group: no change in normal habits for 12 months. Measure: Beck Depression Inventory (BDI).	(+) Regardless of program assignment, greater exercise participation was significantly related to less anxiety and fewer depressive symptoms independent of changes in fitness and body weight.
McMurdo and Rennie (1993); 49 older adults ages 64 to 91. Volunteers from local authority homes, except those with severe communication problems.	Randomized into 2 groups. Exercise: all exercises performed seated. Most exercise consisted of upper and lower limb strengthening to music. Reminiscence sessions to promote social interaction. Both groups participated for 45 min, 2 weeks, 7 months. 3 dropouts. Measure: Geriatric Depression Scale.	(+) Both groups decreased in depression rating. Exercise group showed significantly greater declines than reminiscence group.
Gitlin et al. (1992); 267 older adults (64% F, 36% M), avg. age = 69 (range 60 to 89). Subjects community residents recruited through senior centers and public announcements. All relatively healthy, not depressed to begin with.	Randomized into 2 groups. Bicycle group: 40 min, 3 times/week, 4 months at 70% max HR. Attention group: met in small groups once/week, seminars on "positive lifestyles." 95% completed the 4-month program. Measures: Center for Epidemiology Studies Depression Scale (CES-D). (Radloff, 1977), Affect Balance Scale.	(−) No significant change in depression; significant perceptions of improvement. No significant change in positive or negative affect.

(Continued)

Table 4-3
(*Continued*)

Researchers and sample	Design, treatment, and measures	Findings
Blumenthal et al. (1991); 101 older (50 M, 51 F), avg. age = 67 (range 60 to 83). Healthy sedentary volunteers.	Randomized to 3 groups for 4 months of either: Aerobic: 3 times/week for 30 min; Yoga: twice/week for 60 min; Wait list control. After 4 months all subjects performed aerobic exercise, 12 dropouts. Measures: Centre for Epidemiological Studies Depression Scale (CES-D).	(+ n.s.) Trend toward reduced depression with exercise; however these results did not reach significance.
McNeil et al. (1991); 30 older adults, avg. age = 72.5. Subjects were depressed elderly. No cognitive impairments, not receiving treatment for emotional problems; would participate in any group.	Randomized into 3 groups. Walking group: 20 to 40 min at 3 times week (2 walks were with psych student) for 6 weeks. Walking was vigorous but not overtaxing. Social group: 2 home visits per week with psych student, 20 to 40 min. No dropouts. Measure: Beck Depression Inventory (BDI; Beck & Beamesderfer, 1974).	(+) Both exercise and social group had significant reductions in the total scores and psychological scores (of BDI) as compared to control. The exercise group however, also decreased somatic symptoms of the BDI.
Emery and Gatz (1990); 48 older adults (40 F, 8 M), avg. age = 72 (range 61 to 86). Sedentary, ethnically diverse, volunteers, 80% no education beyond high school; mostly low- and middle-income.	Randomized to aerobic exercise, social activity, or waiting list groups. Aerobic group: 3 times/week for 12 weeks, reaching 70% max HR. Social group: met 3 times/week for 12 weeks for nonphysical activity. 39 of 48 completed 12-week program (19% attrition). Measure: CES-Depression.	(−) No significant change in psychological well-being including depression. Researchers noted that the exercise intervention may have been insufficient; apparently healthy mood scores were already optimal.

(*Continued*)

Table 4-3
(*Continued*)

Researchers and sample	Design, treatment, and measures	Findings
Blumenthal et al. (1989); 101 older adults (51 F, 50 M), avg. age = 67 (range 60 to 83). Healthy but sedentary volunteers.	Randomized to 3 groups for 4 months. Aerobic: 3 times/week for 30 min. Yoga: twice per week for 60 min. Control group. 97 completed study. Measure: CES-Depression.	(+) Significantly reduced depression among males in aerobic group. No significant results for any other group.
Minor et al. (1989); 120 older adults. Subjects had either rheumatoid arthritis (RA), avg. age = 54 yrs, or osteoarthritis (OA), avg. age = 63 yrs. Recruited from clinics.	Subjects assigned to one of three groups: Aerobic walking; aerobic aquatics, range of motion (ROM), control group. All subjects met for 1 hour, 3 times/week, for 12 weeks. Walking and aquatic groups exercised at 60% to 80% of max HR. Five dropouts. Measures: Arthritis Impact Measurement Scale (AIMS) - Anxiety subscales of AIMS.	(+) Significant changes for depression and anxiety reduction for exercise groups over control groups. Aerobic and fitness measures showed significant improvement.
Gayle et al. (1988); 15 older adults (6 F, 9 M) ages 46 to 71. (COPD) patients.	Randomized into 2 groups: 9 experimental, 6 controls. Experimental: 2 consecutive exercise periods, 50/min 3 times/week, for 14 weeks. Pre/post and halfway testing. Controls did not participate in initial 14-week exercise program. 1 dropout at 1st assessment; 2 more dropouts at 2nd assessment. Measure: Zung Self-Rating Depression Scale.	(+ n.s.) Slight nonsignificant reductions; too few subjects; anecdotal comments supported mood improvement.

(*Continued*)

Table 4-3

(*Continued*)

Researchers and sample	Design, treatment, and measures	Findings
Martinsen et al. (1985); 43 older adults, avg. age = 40 (range 17 to 60). Hospitalized patients with depression. Psychotic and patients with physical constraints excluded.	Subjects randomly assigned to exercise or control group. Patients exercised for 9 weeks, 3 sessions/week, for an hour at a time, at 50% to 70% of maximum aerobic capacity. Control group attended occupational therapy. Measure: Beck Depression Inventory.	(+) Significant reduction in depression scores for exercise group, with a corresponding significant increase in aerobic power compared to control group. Supports claims that mildly depressed individuals can benefit from exercise.
Vallient and Asu (1985); 114 older adults ages 50 to 80. Volunteers.	Four groups (nonrandom). Structured exercise: biweekly, 60 min, for 12 weeks. Calisthenics and flexibility exercises. Self-imposed exercise: ongoing involvement in self-regulated activities. Social: participated in ongoing social activities. Controls. Measure: Minnesota Multiphasic Personality Depression Scale.	(+) Significant differences between self-imposed exercisers and social groups. Elderly people who were more fearful, depressed, and assertive appeared to more driven to seek out exercise as a means of reducing these states.
Dustman et al. (1984); 43 elders (27 M, 16 F); avg. age = 60.1 (range 55 to 70). Sedentary, individuals screened for good health.	Randomized for aerobic exercise or strength and flexibility. Non-randomized no-exercise control group. Aerobic: 1 hour, 3 times/week for 4 months (increasing HR to 70% to 80% max). Strength: 1 hour, 3 times/week for 4 months (HR < 70% Max). Measures: Beck Depression Index, Self-Rating Depression Scale.	(−) No significant change as a result of exercise. This was attributed to normal mood levels at the start of the study.

(*Continued*)

Table 4-3
(*Continued*)

Researchers and sample	Design, treatment, and measures	Findings
Perri and Templar (1984/1985); 42 older adults (28 F, 14 M); avg. age = 65 (ages 60 to 79), volunteers.	Nonrandomized controls. Exercise consisted of walking-jogging exercise: 30 min aerobic (40% to 50% of max effort), 3 times/week for 14 weeks. Control group maintained current lifestyle. 17 dropouts. Measure: Zung Self-Rating Depression Scale.	(+) Significant improvement on depression scores for exercise group.

Studies focused on nondepressed subjects have increasingly failed to find any significant effect of exercise on depression. Of the recent studies, which used more rigorous methodologies than many earlier studies, only Blumenthal et al. (1989) and King et al. (1993) found a significant effect of exercise in samples from populations who were not clinically depressed.

Blumenthal et al. (1989) found significantly reduced depression scores in elderly adults after 4 months of aerobic exericse or yoga, but only in the male exercisers in their study. Three studies, Blumenthal et al. (1991), Dustman et al. (1984), and Emery and Gatz (1990), provided evidence which challenges the claims that exercise causes significant reductions in depression among the elderly. A second study by Blumenthal et al. (1991) was a continuation of the above-mentioned 1989 study, where the same subjects participated in an additional 10 months of exercise. Correlations between changes in aerobic power (peak VO_2) and changes in psychological functioning were small and not statistically significant.

Research has been conducted with hospitalized patients (Blankfort-Doyle, 1989; Molloy et al., 1988) and highly anxious elderly (deVries & Adams, 1972). Although significant improvements in cognitive performances were found, Molloy et al. (1988) failed to find any effect on depression. Similar results were shown by Blankfort-Doyle et al. (1989) in their research on impaired nursing home residents. However, the exercise intervention may have been ineffective since Blankfort-Doyle et al. (1989) failed to change any physiological or functional levels of the subjects. However, aerobic fitness may not be necessary if psychological benefits can be obtained from mental and physical relaxation activities. Finally, Gayle et al. (1988) found there were declines in depression with exercise in working with chronic obstructive pulmonary disease (COPD) patients.

Several correlational studies cited in Table 4-4 found that increased levels of physical activity were associated with reduced levels of depression (Kaplan et al., 1993; Krause et al., 1993; Weaver & Narsavage, 1992; Lobstein et al., 1989; Stephens, 1988). Particularily convincing is the work of Stephens (1988), whose study consisted of analyzing data from four national surveys. While direct mechanisms cannot be understood from this research, it seems that those people who maintain an active lifestyle are less likely to become depressed. Whether psychologically healthy individuals are simply more physically active, or whether participation in activities makes individuals more psychologically healthy, still remains unknown.

Some research has suggested that there may not need to be an increase in aerobic fitness for individuals in aerobic programs to experience reduced depression (McMurdo & Rennie, 1993). Participation in an exercise program can elicit a reduction in depression, regardless of an increase in aerobic capacity. However other depression research has suggested that exercise intensity level is important (McNeil et al., 1991). For example, healthy non-depressed individuals may become irritable and depressed as a result of high training loads (e.g., Hatfield et al., 1987).

SELF-ESTEEM OUTCOMES

Summary

Evidence for a relationship between self-esteem and exercise among older adults is **inconclusive**. Little research has been done on the relationship between exercise and self-esteem among elderly populations.

Self-esteem is usually defined as the evaluative aspect of the self (i.e., how the individual feels about his/her perceived self). Individuals can have positive or negative reactions to their perceived characteristics. Self-esteem is most commonly understood (in the research literature) as a hierarchical structure, with global self-esteem at the apex, and physical, social, and other types of self-esteem below. As such, research measuring only global esteem may not be sensitive enough to capture possible changes in physical self-esteem scores.

Correlational research suggests that people with a history of active living and current involvement in physical activity have a higher self-esteem. These studies do not necessarily support causality. For institutionalized populations there is some evidence to support the notion that exercise may increase self-esteem. It

Table 4-4

Depression Outcomes: Correlational and Epidemiological Studies

Researchers and sample	Measures	Findings
Kaplan et al. (1993); 356 older adults ages 65 and over. Representative of non-institutionalized elderly population. 6-year study. 152 were lost as a result of death, could not be located, or declined to be interviewed.	Self-reported exercise participation scales. MMPI-Depression. ADL Functional Scales (Kaplan et al., 1993).	(+) Depression was significantly associated with declines in functioning. (Health is a confound).
Krause et al. (1993); 2,200 older, 60+ years, Nationwide survey of older adults in Japan. One point in time survey.	Self-reported exercise patterns. Centre for Epidemiological Studies Depression Scale.	(+) More frequent exercise is associated with less psychological distress.
Weaver and Narsavage (1992); 104 older adults ages 40 to 84 (avg. age = 65.5). Convenience sample 104 COPD outpatients. Diagnosed for avg. of 11.6 years; 48% < high school education; 82% male; 92% Caucasian; 70% married; 76% unemployed; one point in time survey.	Exercise capacity-12 min walk. Multiple Affect Adjective Check List Revised (MAACL-R). Functional Status Scale (Weaver & Narsavage, 1989).	(+) The combined variables of exercise capacity and depression best predict functional status. Small but significant correlations were found.
Lobstein et al. (1989); 220 older adults; all men; ages 40 to 60. Healthy middle-age men. No tobacco, substance abuse; low alcohol use; no prescribed medication. Self-selected as physically active (jogging an average of 20 mi/week for last three years), or sedentary. 4 months between first and second measure.	Grouped by activity level (Active vs. Sedentary). Minnesota Multiphasic Personality Inventory (MMPI)-Depression.	(+) Joggers had significantly lower depression scores than sedentary subjects.

(Continued)

Table 4-4

(Continued)

Researchers and sample	Measures	Findings
Segebartt et al. (1988); 25 older adults aged 70 years and over. Recruited from an independent living center; Caucasian; no chronic disease or cancer, mood-altering drugs.	13 active subjects, avg. age = 80.9; 12 inactive subjects; avg. age = 81.8. Self-reported exercise. Active criteria: average 123 min/week for last 30 years. Inactive reported approx. 69 years of inactivity. Geriatric Depression Scale. Beck Depression Inventory. Profile of Mood States (POMS).	(−) There was no association of depression and an active lifestyle. Small sample sizes.
Stephens (1988); Over 53,000 older adults. All ages. Secondary analysis of 4 surveys: National Health and Nutrition Exam Survey (1971–1975); Canada Health Survey (1978/1979); National Survey of Personal Health Practices and Consequences (1979); Canada Fitness Survey (1981). Cross-sectional.	Physical activity assessed using 4 techniques: single question on recreational activity; 7 questions on frequency of activity; 2-week recall of 15 activities; 104 activities listed for a 12-month recall. Centre for Epidemiological Studies-Depression. Bradburn Affect Balance Scale. Health Opinion Survey.	(+) Level of physical activity was shown to be positively associated with lower levels of depression and mood state; association especially strong for women and people over 40 years of age. Researchers claim that quality of time is more important than mere energy expended in explaining psychological benefits.

seems that those with lower initial self-esteem scores stand to benefit the most from exercise.

Discussion of the Evidence

As noted by McAuley (1991), self-esteem is commonly acknowledged as the psychological variable having the most potential for benefit from physical activity. On the other hand, self-esteem may influence health by encouraging the adoption of other health-related behaviors.

Research with younger adults has found a strong relationship between the variables of exercise and self-esteem (Wankel, 1993). Among younger adults, those most likely to benefit from exercise in terms of increasing self-esteem are those who have poor self-esteem initially. Most studies have recruited healthy volunteers as subjects, and their levels of esteem may already be optimal as indicated by their willingness to engage in a physical measurement study. People with optimal self-esteem are less likely to make significant gains.

The data on elderly adults, physical activity, and self-esteem are very limited. Volden et al. (1990) sampled 478 adults (ages 18 to 74) across a spectrum of variables, such as rural-urban location, gender, and age. No significant differences were found in self-esteem using the Rosenberg Self-Esteem Scale across the various age groups. The self-esteem scores in this study were high and were attributed to the high levels of education, but women exhibited significantly lower self-esteem scores than men.

Valliant & Asu (1985) examined the differences of structured and unstructured exercisers, along with a social group (activities in a social setting) and a control group in 114 adults between 50 and 80 years of age. There were no significant differences in self-esteem between any of the groups despite reduced depression scores.

Duffy and MacDonald (1990) found a clustering of self-esteem and exercise with current health status. Their findings are similar to those of Hawkins et al. (1988), as well as Ostrow and Dzewaltowski (1986), showing that higher self-esteem and internal locus of control were significantly related to a life span history of exercising as well as current involvement.

Weaver and Narsavage (1992) found in their research on COPD patients that self-esteem was positively correlated with functional status and negatively correlated with depression. As such, increasing functional status (possibly through active living) for these patients may be important for increasing self-esteem. Finally, Perri and Templar (1984/1985), in their fourteen-week aerobic exercise program on older adults, found significant increases in self-concept.

Table 4-5 summarizes intervention and comparison studies of physical activity and self-esteem; Table 4-6 summarizes correlational and epidemiological studies.

BODY IMAGE OUTCOMES

Summary

The level of evidence for a relationship between physical activity participation and body image is **suggestive for women** but **weak for men**. Little research has been

Table 4-5
Self-Esteem Outcomes: Intervention and Comparison Studies

Researchers and sample	Design, treatment, and measures	Findings
Loomis and Thomas (1991); 53 older adults, all women. All subjects needed less than 1.5 hours of professional care per day. One interview.	Two groups of elderly women: 25 nursing home residents (avg. age = 79.8); 28 independent living in own home (avg. age = 68.9). Independent elderly are assumed to take part in more activities of daily living. Measure: Index of Self-Esteem (ISE).	(−) No significant difference in reported self-esteem for nursing home residents and independent living residents (an indirect assumption of active living).
Volden et al. (1990); 478 older adults (291 M, 187 F); avg. age = 40 (range 18 to 74). Convenience sample urban and rural. Survey questionnaire. 478 of 524 surveys returned.	Three sample groups: Nonexercisers; Recent exercisers (less than 6 months); Long-time exercisers (> 7 months). Self-reported exercise using the Health-Promoting Lifestyle Profile (HPLP), Rosenberg Self-Esteem Scale.	(−) Self-esteem was not related significantly to exercise participation.
Perri & Templar (1985). 42 older adults (28 F, 14 M); avg. age = 65 (range 60 to 79). Volunteers.	Two groups (nonrandom assignment). Exercise: (40% to 50% of max effort); 30 min of aerobic exercise (walking and jogging) 3 times/wk for 14 weeks. Control group maintained current lifestyle for 14 weeks. 17 dropouts. Measure: Tennessee Self-Concept Scale.	(+) There was a significant increase in self-concept in the elderly exercising group.

(*Continued*)

Table 4-5
(Continued)

Researchers and sample	Design, treatment, and measures	Findings
Valliant and Asu (1985); 114 older adults; ages 50 to 80. Volunteers.	Four nonrandom groups: Structured exerciser participants; Structured program: twice/week, 60 min, for 12 weeks; calisthenics and flexibility exercises. Self-imposed exercisers; ongoing involvement in self-regulated activities; social group; participated in ongoing social activities; nonexercisers. Measures: no measures of aerobic change. Coppersmith Self-Esteem Inventory.	(−) There were no significant differences in self-esteem in any of the groups.

conducted on the effects of physical activity participation on the body perception of older adults (Hallinan & Schuler, 1993). Even the studies reviewed here have combined middle-age and older adults. However, the results of these few studies have been promising regarding the potential of physical activity to enhance body image.

Tucker and Mortell (1993), in their study of middle-age women, found that those who have the poorest body image to begin with benefit the most. Furthermore, King et al. (1989) found that most benefits accrue within the first month of participation (although their program was quite intensive at five days per week). Both of these studies examined participants who had previously been sedentary.

Discussion of the Evidence

For women at least, body image concerns may persist until at least age 80. In the Hallinan and Schuler (1993) study, exercising women showed a greater discrepancy between their present and ideal shape than nonexercising women did. The authors suggested that women concerned about body shape might self-select into exercise programs. There is also the question of whether group exercise participation invites unfavorable comparisons of one's own body shape with others'. Prospective research on previously sedentary women randomly assigned to exercise alone, exercise in a group, and no exercise at all might help ascertain whether

Table 4-6
Self-Esteem Outcomes: Correlational and Epidemiological Studies

Researchers and sample	Measures	Findings
Weaver and Narsavage (1992); 104 older adults (20 F, 84 M), ages 40 to 84 (avg. age = 65.5). Convenience sample COPD outpatients, diagnosed avg. 11.6 years; 48% < high school; 82% male; 92% Caucasian; 70% married; 76% unemployed.	Exercise capacity: 12-min walk. Rosenberg Self-Esteem Scale. Functional Status Scale (Weaver & Narsavage, 1992).	(+) Self-esteem was significantly correlated with functional status. Self-esteem and depression negatively correlated. Positive association between functional status and exercise.
Duffy & MacDonald (1990); 161 older adults (98 F, 63 M); ages 65 to 99 (avg. age = 74.1 yrs). Purposive sample; 76% Caucasian; 69% widowed, single or divorced; 55% ≤ high school. Median annual income $8,400. One 2-hour interview.	Demographic variables. Rosenberg Self-Esteem Scale (RSE).	(+) Active men had lower incomes, higher internal locus of control, higher self-esteem, more exercise, and better current health status. Exercise and nutrition may be critical health promotion activities — associated with better scores on 5 functional dimensions.

participation in various forms of physical activity would have positive benefits for the body image of older women.

Body image is often seen as a female issue and thus data on males are lacking. There are societal pressures on women (e.g., through the media) to maintain "beauty" (usually defined as thinness and youthful physical attractiveness) as they age. It is unclear how older women may differ from younger women in beliefs about what makes a physically attractive body. Research is also needed on how men feel about their aging bodies (e.g., diminishing muscle size and strength) and whether these concerns can be alleviated through participation in physical activity.

Table 4-7
Body Image Outcomes: Intervention and Comparison Studies

Researchers and sample	Design, treatment, and measures	Findings
Hallinan and Schuler (1993); 78 women; avg. age = 72.6 (range 60 to 88). Volunteer; intervention subjects from adult fitness program, comparison subjects from local community service groups.	49 intervention subjects; 29 comparison subjects. Fitness classes: 3 times/week; intensity, duration not reported. Comparison subjects did no activity. Measured body shape perception. (Stunkard et al. silhouette-scale). Women rated selves on a visual scale from very thin to very heavy. Rated actual and ideal body shape. Group discrepancy examined.	(−) Active women reported a larger discrepancy between current and ideal shape than inactive women; no significant interaction with age, but trend to smaller discrepancy after age 80.
Tucker and Mortell (1993); 65 women; avg. age = 42.9 (range 35 to 49). Sedentary, less than 20% over ideal weight (Metropolitan Life height-weight tables); recruited by newspaper ads in Utah; no chronic health problems or risk factors.	Randomly assigned to weight training or walking (30 subjects per group); 12-week program, 3 times/week. One mile 1st 3 weeks (65% max HR), 2 miles wks 4 to 8 (70% max HR), 2.5 miles wks 9 to 12 (80% max HR). Weight training: Body Bar (attached to bench with elastic cords). Individualized programs; 3 sets of 10 reps for each exercise; moderate intensity first 2 weeks, maximum intensity remaining weeks. Measure: Body Cathexis Scale; women evaluated appearance of selected body parts.	(+) Both exercise groups scored higher on Body Cathexis Scale after than before program. Weight training increased self-esteem more than walking group. Subjects with lowest preprogram scores gained most in body cathexis. Improved body cathexis corresponded to strength improvements for weight training group, and perceived walking intensity at end-program for walking group.

(Continued)

Table 4-7

(*Continued*)

Researchers and sample	Design, treatment, and measures	Findings
King et al. (1989); 120 older adults (60 F, 60 M); avg. age = 47 for women, 49 for men. Sedentary employees of Lockheed Missile and Space Corporation in Sunnyvale, CA. 75% hourly, 25% salaried. No activity-limiting conditions or chronic diseases.	Random assignment to exercise and control groups. Exercise: 6-week home-based and staff-monitored aerobics program (brisk walking or slow jogging). Duration of sessions: avg. 54 min for women, 47 min for men; 5 times/week at 65% to 77% of peak baseline treadmill heart rate. Portable heart monitor. Training frequency, duration, and intensity remained above 75% (on average) of prescribed levels. 57/60 of exercise subjects and 56/60 control subjects completed study. Measures: satisfaction with physical shape and appearance, satisfaction with current body weight.	(+) Exercisers reported significant changes in both types of satisfaction compared to controls. Most changes occurred in first month of program. Satisfaction with weight and shape/physical appearance were correlated. Actual weight loss small for both groups, but satisfaction with weight and actual weight loss were correlated. For women, satisfaction with both weight and shape/appearance were correlated with increased fitness ratings. Satisfaction with weight and shape/appearance also correlated positively with improved mental health (less anxiety, depression).

Finally, the studies cited here have focused on vigorous, prescriptive exercise. It is not known at this point what the benefits of more moderate physical activities might be for body image in older adults. Table 4-7 summarizes the studies reviewed.

LOCUS OF CONTROL OUTCOMES

Summary

The level of evidence for the relationship between physical activity and locus of control is **weak**. Locus of control refers to an individual's perceived influence in regulating life outcomes, based on past experiences which operantly condition people to expect certain outcomes from their actions (Rotter, 1966). Locus of control is expressed as a continuum with a group of individuals demonstrating a range of perceived control from "internality" to "externality."

Health locus of control has been defined as perceived control over one's health. An internal locus of control is the perception that health outcomes are a result of individual actions, whereas an external locus of control is the perception that health outcomes are related to chance, external factors, or the actions of others (Kist-Kline, 1989; Wallston & Wallston, 1978). Locus of control has been conceptualized as having a hierarchical structure, with global locus of control having a relatively permanent trait while the more specific health locus of control may be influenced by personal health and functional status.

Theoretically, positive associations are expected between physical activity and locus of control, as increased mastery from participation is hypothesized to lead to a greater sense of control over the surrounding environment. Some current evidence suggests that increased physical activity may shift locus of control from an external orientation toward an internal orientation, implying that people feel a greater sense of control over their bodies and health. This is most evident in those who initially have an external orientation and who are more sedentary. Health locus of control is more likely to change than the more general locus of control, which is not surprising given that physical activity is widely seen as a health-promoting behavior.

Discussion of the Evidence

Greendale et al. (1993) examined the use of weighted vests as a resistance-type of intervention protocol on independent-living older adults. After the intervention, the subjects using vests experienced a shift in their health locus of control in an internal direction and exhibited higher scores on internal locus of control and lower scores on 'powerful other' and 'chance' subscales in comparison to the controls. The final scores were significantly different on the powerful others and chance scales. While these results have been criticized for methodological problems, Perri and Templar (1984–1985) also found that 42 elderly adults in a 14-week walking/jogging program did enhance locus of control significantly.

Emery and Gatz (1990) studied a 12-week exercise program for an ethnically diverse older population to examine the relationship between exercise, improved internal locus of control and personal mastery. The researchers expected elderly populations to have increases similar to younger populations, who show increases in locus of control or mastery as a result of exercise. Their results showed no significant main effect for the variable of locus of control or mastery with exercise.

Valliant and Asu (1985) studied a self-selected sample of 114 adults, ages 50 to 80. The sample was divided into four categories:

(a) structured exercisers (who followed an exercise program designed by researchers),
(b) self-imposed exercisers,
(c) a social group, and
(d) nonexercisers.

Although they did not investigate causality, it was predicted that lower depression, higher self-esteem, and greater locus of control scores would be reflected by those individuals in physical activity programs. However the results failed to show any significant relationship between exercise participation and locus of control.

In a correlation study, O'Brien Cousins (1993) found internal locus of control was associated with leisure-time physical activity level in a study of 327 Vancouver women over the age of 70. While internality was associated with higher activity level, health locus of control was not a significant predictor of late-life exercise behavior compared to other self-referent constructs such as self-efficacy to exercise and perceived social support to exercise.

While evidence from intervention studies is currently divided, the correlational research is indicative of an association. From their results of 297 volunteers recruited from health fairs, seniors' centers and retirement groups, Speake et al. (1991) found significant relationships between internal locus of control and exercise (along with other positive health behaviors). Individuals with a stronger external locus of control participated in fewer health-related behaviors. Kaplan et al. (1993) also provided support in finding significant associations between locus of control and physical functioning for seniors.

Although the evidence remains mixed, theoretical understanding of behavior would suggest that there is some association between exercise and locus of control. People who are exercising for the purpose of obtaining or maintaining health benefits must first believe that they can personally influence their health through their activity behavior (O'Brien Cousins, 1996). While the results of the intervention studies are mixed, the results of Greendale et al. (1993) (the most methodologically sound) suggested that there is some correlation between exercise and locus of control.

O'Brien Cousins (1993, 1996) has suggested two potential explanations for the ambiguous findings. First, many older people may be exercising for reasons other than controlling their health. For example, older adults may be active mainly for social reasons and to improve their physical appearance. Second, in the O'Brien Cousins study, further analysis revealed a nonlinear relationship between health

Table 4-8
Locus of Control Outcomes: Intervention and Comparison Studies

Researchers and sample	Design, treatment, and measures	Findings
Greendale et al. (1993); 36 older adults (30 F, 6 M); ages 58 to 80. Volunteers from senior center. Excluded for: heart problems; several other physical disorders.	Random assignment to 2 groups: 19 in exercise group, 17 controls. Exercise group: weighted vests, after first 2 weeks wore them at home. Discussion group: led by experts on health education. Both groups met for 1 hour each week for 20 weeks; 5 dropouts. Measures: Multidimensional Health Locus of Control (Wallston & Wallston, 1978); consists of 3 sub-scales: Internal Locus of Control; Chance Locus of Control; Powerful Others Locus of Control.	(+) Exercise subjects reported a statistically significant shift toward internal locus of control. The discussion group tended toward increased externality over time.
Emery and Gatz (1990); 48 older adults (40 F, 8 M); ages 61 to 86 (avg. age = 72). Sedentary, ethnically diverse, volunteers; 80% no education beyond high school, predominately low- and middle-income.	Randomly assigned to aerobic or social activity for 12 weeks. Aerobic: 3 times/ week reaching 70% max HR. Social: met 3 times/week for nonphysical activity. 10 dropouts (wanted to be in exercise group). Measures: Rotter Internal-External Scale; Pearlin Mastery Scale; Lau and Ware Health Locus of Control Scale.	(−) No significant changes in locus of control for exercise group.
Perri and Templar (1984–1985); 42 older adults (28 F, 14 M), ages 60 to 79, avg. age = 65. Volunteers.	Exercise: walking-jogging for 14 weeks; 30 min aerobic (40% to 50% of max effort), 3 times/week. Control group (nonrandom) maintained current lifestyle. 17 dropouts. Measure: Rotter's Locus of Control Scale.	(+) Significant increase in internal locus of control, perhaps indicating an increase in perceived mastery of environment.

(Continued)

Table 4-8
(*Continued*)

Researchers and sample	Design, treatment, and measures	Findings
Valliant and Asu (1985); 114 older adults, ages 50 to 80. Volunteers.	Sample divided into four groups (nonrandom assignment): Structured exercisers: supervised intervention; 12-week program of supervised calisthenics and flexibility exercises. Self-imposed exercisers: ongoing involvement in self-regulated activities. Social group: participate in ongoing social activities; 12-week program of ongoing social activities. Structured program: was biweekly for 60 min. Nonexercisers control group. Measures: Rotter's Locus of Control Inventory. No measures of aerobic change.	(−) No significant difference between the four groups.

and activity behavior: that is, the elderly women with low HLoc who were taking 4 or 5 prescription medications were as physically active as the women with high HLoc who reported good to excellent health and were taking no medications at all. These may be among the reasons why no clear-cut relationship between health locus of control and activity behavior has been found in older adults. Also, self-selection and small samples limit any conclusions which can be drawn from the research in this area.

Table 4-8 presents intervention and comparison studies regarding physical activity and locus of control; Table 4-9 presents correlational and epidemiological studies.

LIFE SATISFACTION OUTCOMES

Summary

The level of evidence for a relationship between physical activity and life satisfaction is **weak**. Life satisfaction is sometimes used as an indicator of perceived quality of life, and is usually measured by the 18-item Life Satisfaction Index.

Table 4-9

Locus of Control Outcomes: Correlational and Epidemiological Studies

Researchers and sample	Measures	Findings
Kaplan et al. (1993); 356 older adults, 65 and over. Representive of non-institutionalized elderly population. 6-year study, 152 subjects were lost as a result to death, could not be located, or declined to be interviewed.	Self-reported exercise participation scales. MMPI-Locus of Control. ADL Functional Scales.	(+) Health locus of control (externality) was significantly associated with declines in functioning.
O'Brien Cousins (1993). 327 women ages 70+; volunteers from seniors' centers, facilities randomly selected in metro Vancouver.	Self-reported weekly exercise (Older Adult Exercise Status Inventory) and health beliefs including health locus of control (HLOC), social support, efficacy for fitness exercise, perceived risks and benefits, and health motive.	(+) Internal HLOC was positively associated with an active lifestyle. (−) HLOC was a weak predictor of late-life exercise compared to other cognitive factors.
Speake et al. (1989); 297 older adults, avg. age = 71.9 (range 55 to 93). Volunteers from health fairs, seniors' centers, and retirement groups in northern Florida. 70.5% female; 54.6 unmarried; 71% Caucasian; 53% with more than high school education. One reporting session.	Self-reported locus of control, perceived health status, and healthy lifestyle as assessed by the Health Promoting Lifestyle Profile. Multidimensional Health Locus of Control. 3 subscales: Internal Locus of Control (IHLC); Chance Locus of Control (CHLC); Powerful Others Locus of Control (PHLC).	(+) Externality (powerful others locus of control) was significantly associated with exercise, possibly indicating that physicians, nurses, and health professionals may influence exercise of the elderly.

Some studies show a strong relationship between increases in leisure participation and increases in life satisfaction. However, few studies since the MacNeil review (1988) have focused on this issue, and none have implemented MacNeil's recommendations to conduct studies over a period of time with individuals at different life stages. In addition, more research is needed to determine which physical activities have a greater influence on life satisfaction. Finally, research should consider how the relationship between physical activity and life satisfaction may differ with sex, education, social class, and health.

Discussion of the Evidence

Much of the focus on the physical activity-life satisfaction relationship was done in the early 1980s, and the studies done by Ragheb and Griffith (1982) and Riddick and Daniel (1984) serve as good benchmarks. A review article by MacNeil (1988) did not mention Emrich's (1985) study on older sports enthusiasts, but the findings corresponded to the conclusions of Steinkamp and Kelly (1987). The only study done in the 1990s was that of Loomis and Thomas (1991), but it did not examine the direct effect of physical activity on life satisfaction.

There is a significant relationship between increases in leisure participation and increases in life satisfaction (Riddick & Daniel, 1984). Riddick and Daniel found that increased leisure participation correlated with increased life satisfaction, and that leisure participation was the strongest contributor to life satisfaction among older women. Leisure satisfaction contributed much more to the life satisfaction of seniors than did simple leisure participation (Ragheb & Griffith, 1982). This coincides with three other studies referenced in MacNeil's (1988) review. These studies found that the social bonding dimension of leisure is central, and that specific activities like sport and exercise take on a lower priority as adults age.

MacNeil concluded in his review (1988) that research up to the mid-1980s had used traditional cross-sectional, descriptive techniques using age as a variable to determine leisure patterns. MacNeil recommended that future research should consider the issue (of leisure participation) from the lifestyle or life-stage approach. Lifestyle and/or life stage may be a more reliable predictor of leisure patterns than chronological age. There also needs to be increased emphasis on longitudinal research.

Life satisfaction is conceivably tied in closely with health status and demographic factors such as sex, social status, education, and work status. Studies to date do not assess or account for these confounding variables in their statistical analyses.

Table 4-10 contains correlational and epidemiological studies. No intervention and comparison studies were reviewed, thus we have no information on causality.

Table 4-10

Life Satisfaction Outcomes: Correlational and Epidemiological Studies

Researchers and sample	Measures	Findings
Kelly et al. (1987); 400 adults > 40, range 40 to 89 (40 to 54 = 40% of sample; 55+ = 60%; 65+ = 30%; > 75 = 10%). Table of random digits of telephone directory in Peoria, Illnois.	Telephone interview followed by intensive interviews. 6-item LSI (life satisfaction index); leisure activity - 4 point scale for 28 categories including sport/exercise.	(+) For adults > 65, leisure as a set of engagements or activities is a significant predictor of life satisfaction; kinds of participation associated with subjective satisfaction were travel, cultural, and social activities, then exercise/sport, followed by outdoor, family, and home-based activities.
Emrich (1985); German abstract in *Sportunterricht* *34*(9): 341–346. Abstract only available. Avg. age = 75. Senior citizens, thus assumed > 65; sports enthusiasts.	Level of activity, perceived life satisfaction.	(+) A high level of activity was positively correlated with perceived life satisfaction.
Riddick & Daniel (1984); 1,101 women ages 65 and over (avg. age = 73, 698 retirees) 403 homemakers; secondary database.	Leisure activities index: social life, media, leisure, recreation (including walking and sports), organizations, and voluteer work; employment status; health problems; income. Life satisfaction index (18 items).	(+) Strong association between leisure participation and life satisfaction, leisure participation strongest contributor to life satisfaction among older women. Significant relationship between increases in leisure participation and increases in life satisfaction; retirees participated in leisure activities more frequently than homemakers. Income had the strongest indirect effect on life satisfaction via its influence on participation in leisure activities.

KNOWLEDGE, BELIEF, AND ATTITUDE OUTCOMES

Summary

The level of evidence for a relationship between physical activity and knowledge, beliefs and attitudes is **weak**. Very little research has examined knowledge, beliefs, or attitudes as *outcomes* of participation in physical activity by older adults. Most research has examined these variables as predictors of involvement in physical activity (e.g., Sharpe & Connell, 1992; Ferrini et al., 1994; Fitzgerald et al., 1994) or correlates (e.g., Jones et al., 1992). There is some evidence that participation in a program positively influences attitudes among older adults, but there were too few older subjects to examine for age-specific results (Steinhardt & Young, 1992).

Discussion of the Evidence

Models such as the Health Belief Model (Becker, 1974) and the Theory of Reasoned Action/Planned Behavior (Ajzen, 1985; 1991), argue that knowledge, beliefs, and attitudes precede behavioral choices. Although such models do not deny a reciprocal effect of behavior on cognition and affect, they emphasize behavior as the main dependent variable. It is therefore not surprising that research guided by such models would focus on attitudes or beliefs as predictors, but not outcomes, of participation in physical activity. Most exercise researchers tend to view exercise outcomes as changes in physical or mental health status. The use of physical activity interventions to reinforce knowledge, beliefs, and attitudes has not been given much attention. Self-efficacy is somewhat of an exception (see next section).

One study that did examine attitudes as an outcome of physical activity is Shephard et al. (1986). They studied 86 randomly selected (46 F, 40 M) 45 to 75-year-old employees and former employees of the University of Toronto. Participants were randomly assigned to one of three groups: health education, exercise plus health education, or control group. The health education condition consisted of a once per week lecture and discussion on exercise, obesity control, and smoking. The exercise plus health education condition met once per week, with one hour of progressive endurance exercise (with emphasis on movement education), followed by lecture/discussion as above. Participants in this group were also given an exercise prescription, based on fitness testing, to do on their own four times week. Both programs lasted 20 weeks. Fifty-two (60.5%) of subjects completed the whole program; (10 health education; 21 health education plus exercise; 21 controls). Outcomes were

(a) attitudes toward the instrumental value of exercise: socializing, aesthetic activity, ascetic activity, pursuit of vertigo, tension release, health and fitness, games of chance (Kenyon, 1968), and

(b) health attitudes assessed by the Cornell Medical Index. No significant differences in pre- and post-program scores were found.

However, an earlier study (Sidney & Shephard, 1976) had found participants aged 60 and over in a program of four one hour classes per week did change their scores on the Kenyon instrument. It is not clear whether the narrower age range of the participants in the earlier study or the more structured nature of the intervention accounted for the differences in results.

Most studies that have examined "attitudes" as outcomes do not use measures that clearly separate attitude from other psychological constructs. For instance, the items on the Kenyon scale, which measure the extent to which respondents believe exercise provides a means to certain ends, is closer to the outcome belief construct (e.g., Ajzen, 1985, 1991). Those theorists define attitude as a more general feeling toward behavior, with both affective (e.g., pleasant-unpleasant) and cognitive (e.g., beneficial-harmful) dimensions. Research on perceived physical activity outcomes is needed which clearly distinguishes between attitudes and beliefs, and beliefs and knowledge. (Knowledge in this context can be viewed as awareness of factual information about a behavior; beliefs as the perception that a behavior has various consequences for oneself.) These distinctions are often made in the literature on predictors of physical activity.

SELF-EFFICACY OUTCOMES

Summary

The level of evidence for a relationship between physical activity and self-efficacy among older adults is **suggestive**, mainly because there have been few studies to date. As McAuley et al. (1993) noted, most research on the relationship between physical activity and self-efficacy has examined self-efficacy as a *predictor* of physical activity (see McAuley, 1992 for a review of this research). The limited number of studies that have examined self-efficacy as an *outcome* have found that participation in physical activity positively influences self-efficacy levels in older adults (see Table 4-11). Possible mechanisms are performance-based feedback (through fitness testing) and positive affect during exercise.

The benefits of physical activity regarding self-efficacy seem especially strong for women. However, more studies are needed across a variety of population sub-

Table 4-11

Self-Efficacy Outcomes: Intervention and Comparison Studies

Researchers and sample	Design, treatment, and measures	Findings
McAuley et al. (1993); 82 subjects initially (26F, 18M); avg. age = 44; sedentary for at least 6 mos.; no health problems, volunteer convenience sample, non-random.	Intervention study of 20-week structured classes, 3 times/ week for 1 hr., intensity monitored by instructor. Then exercise on own for next 9 mos. (follow-up), reported frequency, but not intensity. 44 of 82 (53.6%) retested after 9 mos. Of those, 50% reported non-compliance to exercise prescription they were given post-program, 40% reported being nonregular exercisers. Measured self-efficacy for: physical activity (sit-ups, bicycling, walking/jogging); rated confidence for 0% to 100% for each level they felt they could achieve in progressive levels (number of sit-ups, progressive bicycling time periods and workload, walk/jog successive 1/4 miles within 4-min. intervals. Graded exercise testing (GXT).	(+) Bicycle efficacy increased pre- to post-GXT immed. after 20-wk. program; decreased over 9 mos. follow-up; increased again post-GXT (at 9 mos. follow-up) to 20-wk. level. Similar results for sit-up self-efficacy; walking self-efficacy declined over 9 mos. follow-up, and did not rebound post 9 mos. GXT; adherence self-efficacy at 20 weeks predicted exercise maintenance over 9 mos.; no gender differences.
McAuley and Courneya (1992); 88 older adults (46F, 42M). Avg. age = 53.5 (range 45 to 64).	One-time cycle erg. Graded Exercise Test (GXT), modified Astrand-Rhyming. Pedalled to 70% of predicted max heart rate. Self-efficacy for cycling and walking, measured as above; pre- and post-GXT.	(+) Increase in self-efficacy at post-GXT; in-task affect (Feeling Scale) predicted post-GXT self-efficacy.

(*Continued*)

Table 4-11
(Continued)

Researchers and sample	Design, treatment, and measures	Findings
McAuley et al. (1991); 103 subjects (53F, 50M), 81 subjects available for post-GXT. Avg. age = 54.	As in McAuley et al. (1993), but without 9 mos. follow-up. 81 of 103 (78.6%) available for post-GXT. Measures as in McAuley et al. (1993). Females had lower self-efficacy than males prior to program for all three types of activity. Self-efficacy corresponded to actual fitness levels.	(+) Males and females significantly increased self-efficacy pre- to post-GXT at 20 wks. For sit-up efficacy, females' self-efficacy increased over 20 weeks; males' did not.
Oldridge & Rogowski (1990); 76 initially, 51 completed. Total sample 76% M, 23% F. 59 ± 11.2. Discharged patients from intensive or coronary care unit, no contraindications to early ambulation, randomized to conditions, stratified according to ejection fraction, similar in gender, age, weight, race, occupation, reason for referral, and smoking status; patients not assigned to program until they could walk 800 feet.	Two randomly assigned groups no control: 25 exercise center program (treadmill or cycling), 26 ward ambulation program (walking). Daily supervised sessions, intensity limited to HR < 20 bpm above resting HR or 3–4 on perceived exertion scale; exercise center patients progressed to 20–25 min; time not given for ward ambulation. Self-efficacy assessed at 5 points: when consent for randomization obtained, day of discharge from coronary or ICU, day of discharge from hospital, 7 and 28 days after discharge from hospital; scales measured self-reported ability for: walking distance, walking time, climbing stairs, lifting objects, and tolerance for physical exertion.	(+) At 28 days, self-efficacy for walking time and exertion was higher for exercise center patients. For both groups, there was significant increase over course of study in both groups for all physical activities, household activities, daily living tasks, and return to work. Authors suggest that difference between exercise center and ward ambulation was too small to justify expense of the exercise center.

(Continued)

Table 4-11

(*Continued*)

Researchers and sample	Design, treatment, and measures	Findings
Atkins et al. (1984); 76 older adults (48F, 28M); avg. age = 64.8; severe cardiopulmonary obstructive disease patients; half physician-referred, others self-referred; from all SES strata.	Random assignment to one of 5 conditions: behavior modification, cognitive mod, cog-behav mod. attention-only control, no-treatment control. Individualized prescriptions and cognitive and/or behavioral strategies developed with subject to encourage compliance. 5 dropouts total (6.6%). Measure: efficacy expectations re: how far they could walk.	(+) All 3 experimental groups had significantly higher self-efficacy after 3 months compared to attention-only control group.
Hogan and Santomier (1984); 38 older adults; (27 F, 11 M). Avg. age for exercisers = 65.5 for F, 72.3 for M; avg. age for controls 70.6 for F, 67.0 for M. Volunteers, non-institutionalized, healthy, non-random (depending on day and time of their program section).	Two groups (nonrandom): 18 exercisers, 20 controls. Exercise: swim lessons, 5 wks. Once/wk, beginner level; dropout, 3 (15%) from control group. Measure: Swim Skills Efficacy Scale, open-ended question regarding change in feelings about their ability.	(+) Beginner swimmers reported significant change in self-efficacy for swimming at post-test; controls did not. 78% reported positive change in feelings about their ability.

groups (especially age differences) and a variety of physical activities (both structured and less structured).

Discussion of the Evidence

McAuley et al. (1991, 1993) found that women in particular gained in self-efficacy after participating in physical activity. Men started out with higher self-efficacy before a 20-week exercise program, but the gender differences disappeared by post-program as women's self-efficacy increased. They also found that self-efficacy can decrease over the course of a 20-week program (McAuley et al., 1991) or 9-month follow-up (McAuley et al., 1993), then rebound after cycle ergometer and abdominal strength tests. Both the gender by time interaction and the "rebound" effect suggest an important role for performance feedback in influencing self-efficacy. The specificity of self-efficacy was also evident in these studies, as exercise test feedback influenced self-efficacy for cycling and sit-ups, but not for walking/jogging. This is not surprising considering that the exercise tests involved cycle ergometry and abdominal strength, but not walking or jogging.

Only the more recent studies (McAuley et al., 1991, 1993; McAuley & Courneya, 1992; Oldridge & Rogowski, 1990) used the self-efficacy measurement procedures recommended by Bandura (1977). The earlier studies (Hogan & Santomier, 1984; Atkins et al., 1984) used less specific questions. However, both the earlier and later studies supported the notion of a positive influence of physical activity participation on self-efficacy.

More research is needed with larger sample sizes, so that differences among subgroups can be studied. For instance, does physical activity have similar or different influences on self-efficacy for adults in their 50s, 60s, 70s, or 80s? Are there differences among socioeconomic groups? As with most physical activity research, the studies cited here have been with mostly Caucasian, middle-income, well-educated (in terms of formal schooling) people who live in urban centers containing universities. As well, most of the activities have been highly structured classes or other forms of exercise prescription. More study of day-to-day physical activities is needed (i.e., the diversity of active living). Although most of the studies have included both women and men, further study of gender differences is needed across different types of physical activities (in which women and men have different degrees of experience).

More research is needed with different types of programs. Oldridge and Rogowski's finding that two programs for a patient population (exercise center and ward ambulation) led to quite similar results has implications for practitioners planning programs. If two programs appear equal, factors such as user preferences, ease of implementation, and relative program cost, need to be considered.

Perhaps the greatest weakness in this research is the very small number of studies with self-efficacy as an outcome of increased physical activity, rather than as a predictor. In particular, mechanisms by which participation influences self-efficacy need more study. The research discussed here suggests that performance feedback (McAuley et al., 1991, 1993) and positive affect during exercise (McAuley & Courneya, 1992) play important roles.

Table 4-11 illustrates intervention and comparison studies in this area. No correlational or epidemiological studies were reviewed.

Chapter 5

Lifestyle Behavior Outcomes

HABITUAL PHYSICAL ACTIVITY OUTCOMES

Summary

The level of evidence for a relationship between habitual and present physical activity among older adults is **indicative**. Although there is much research addressing adherence in younger adults, the influence of habitual participation in physical activity on present participation among older adults is sparse. A few studies have found that past exercise behavior or even recalled childhood activity predicts current exercise behavior (e.g., Morris et al., 1990; O'Brien Cousins, 1997). However, there is also evidence for discontinuity of leisure-time physical activity in the early adult years. Late-life disruptions in habitual activity patterns may be because of poor health. For example, Drummond (1990) noted that older adults who have experienced a serious illness may severely curtail their activity. Other researchers have suggested that for some people, health problems may act as incentives to increase physical activity (O'Brien Cousins, 1993).

Discussion of the Evidence

There is some longitudinal research that has shown past activity to be correlated with present activity, at least for men. Morris et al. (1990) found that 51 percent of men who were active in vigorous sports, and 19 percent of those active in other vigorous activities in 1976, were still active in 1982–1984. By contrast, among men *inactive* in 1976, the respective percentages were 13 percent and 9.5 percent. The men in their study were British civil servants ages 45 to 64 in 1976. Habitual activity may be important, although there is some evidence (e.g., Paffenbarger et al., 1993) that men taking up physical activity later in life have the same low mortality risk as those who have been active all along.

Very few intervention studies have been conducted to determine if participation in physical activity leads to a continued active lifestyle among older adults (e.g., Hamdorf et al., 1993). Hamdorf et al. found that women in a walking program adopted and maintained a higher level of physical activity compared to a control group. Mayer et al. (1994) found that older adults in a preventive care program (in a health maintenance organization) increased their physical activity relative to those in a regular care program. In addition, more patients in the preventive care program moved from sedentary to active during the 12-months follow-up.

O'Brien Cousins and Keating (1995) found qualitative evidence with women in focus groups which suggests that the life course is disrupted by work patterns, marriage and family responsibilities. However, their findings on "life turning points" suggest that active women tend to adapt to life stage change in physically active ways while sedentary women acknowledge the same life stage features as creating barriers to their personal activity levels. In a separate quantitative research project, O'Brien Cousins (1997) found that women born at the turn of the century (1896 to 1920) who reported high levels of confidence for physical fitness activity at late life were also recalling high efficacy for "tomboy skills" in their girlhood. In multiple regression analysis, both of these efficacy ratings were significantly associated with current physical activity level.

A qualitative study of 10 older adults ages 65 to 76 examined the subjective outcomes of a company-sponsored exercise and fitness program (Rudman, 1987). Subjects reported changes in social, personal, and health habits for the better (smoking cessation, awareness of cholesterol intake, weight reduction). All 10 individuals entered the program because of physical problems with weight, high blood pressure, arthritis, or symptoms of heart disease. Although a number of positive health habit changes were reported as a result of exercise participation, physical activity level outside of the program was not. It may be that the employees felt they were getting sufficient physical activity participation within the program.

Some evidence suggests that older adults may participate outside of an exercise program if the program itself has a low frequency. For example, in a once-per-week Red Cross Fun and Fitness program for older adults, the participants substantially increased their weekly participation in other exercise activities as they got older (Myers & Hamilton, 1985). The program apparently acted as a motivator, catering to inactive but healthy seniors, leading 58 percent of the participants to engage in several other physical activities each week in addition to the Fun and Fitness Program.

Emrich (1989) reported on a qualitative study of the life activity patterns of 75 athletic adults, average age 67. These older athletes had been engaged in sport virtually all of their lives. Positive experiences in school physical education and sport were acknowledged by participants as the important origin of lifelong athletic physical activity.

A pilot study by D'Urso and Logue (1988) involved competitive adapted sports for frail elderly. A competitive volleyball league was established among impaired elderly from adult day health care centers. According to the researchers, the qualitative results were very positive for both participants and volunteers alike. Participants were reported to enjoy this new activity experience, which was believed to fill a void of isolation and relocation with camaraderie and cooperation.

Graham et al. (1992) conducted a study among the older population on spending time in shopping malls. The study determined that a major reason for this was an interest in sociability. Although there were no active living outcomes directly identified, spending time in malls requires basic mobility and offers a potential for seniors to become active in mall-walking clubs.

Researchers and practitioners need to develop a better understanding of the role of developing competency in physical activity in promoting habitual participation. There appears to be a link between perceived competence and movement confidence and physical activity at earlier life stages, and a suggestion that the same is true with older adults. Biographical research would help researchers and practitioners understand the triggers to reinstating involvement in exercise, as well as identifying the sources of disruptions which act as barriers to participation.

The research that has been done has relied mostly on self-report measures of physical activity, and some sample sizes have been small. Several studies included only men or only women, making an analysis of gender differences impossible.

Table 5-1 contains intervention and comparison studies. Table 5-2 contains correlational/epidemiological studies. The qualitative studies are included in Table 5-2 as well, as they involved retrospective recall and perceptions rather than responses to present or recent interventions.

TOBACCO AND ALCOHOL-RELATED OUTCOMES

Summary

The level of evidence for the influence of physical activity on smoking and/or alcohol abuse among older adults is **weak**. Most research on the inter-relationship among lifestyle behaviors has not focused on older adults (see Wankel & Sefton, 1993 for a review).

Table 5-1
Habitual Physical Activity Outcomes: Intervention and Comparison Studies

Researchers and sample	Design, treatment, and measures	Findings
Mayer et al. (1994); 1,922 older adults (1,008 F, 992 M); avg. age = 73.1. Members of a health maintenance organization (HMO). Subjects had relatively high education and income levels, and most reported good health.	Randomly assigned to one of two groups: 899 to preventive care, 901 to regular care. 6-year project with 2-year intervention period. Preventive care included health risk appraisal, goal setting, face-to-face counseling, phone checks on progress; used Growing Wiser, Growing Younger program (8 sessions); with physical activity (three times per week for at least 30 minutes). 84% of preventive care and 88% of regular care group completed the 12-month assessment. 59% attended at least 6 of 8 group sessions. Measured frequency of physical activity outside program. Baseline and 12-month follow-up compared.	(+) Increasing physical activity was most common goal (by 42%). Walking, swimming, and a combination of activities were most popular. Physical activity (aerobic, stretching, strength exercises) increased over time for preventive care group. More preventive than usual care subjects shifted from sedentary to a more active category over the 12 months (24% from 14%).
Hamdorf et al. (1993); 66 subjects (all women), avg. age = 64.8.	Subjects randomly assigned to one of two groups: 30 to walking group, 36 to control group. 26-week progressive walking program, twice per week; breathing hard criteria for intensity. Subjects encouraged to continue physical activity on their own after the program. 90% of walking and 86.1% of control group available for 12-month follow-up. 47.5% combined dropout for 6-month program and follow-up. Measures: Human Activity Profile (highest intensity person can perform), Normative Impairment Index (subtracts activities person cannot do, from highest level).	(+) 77.8% of walking group reported continuing with exercise for the follow-up period. 74.2% of control group reported not starting any regular exercise during the follow-up period. Walking group had significantly higher HAP and NII scores than controls at end of training. Differences were maintained over follow-up period, but scores did not increase.

Table 5-2

Habitual Physical Activity Outcomes: Correlational and Epidemiological Studies

Researchers and sample	Measures	Findings
O'Brien Cousins (1993); 550 women, ages 70 to 98 (avg. age = 77). Community-dwelling women, Vancouver, B.C. Surveyed over 8 months. 327 surveys completed.	10 demographic attributes; 6 cognitive beliefs. Multiple regression analysis to explain late-life exercise (estimated kilo-calories per week of leisure-time physical activity).	(+) Health, childhood involvement, childhood encouragement, cultural background, age were significant predictors explaining 18% of late-life exercise.
Emrich (1989); 75 older adults, avg. age = 67. Athletic seniors. One point in time assessment.	Interviews examining activity level, life satisfaction, biographical and motivational factors. Continuity of lifelong engagement in physical activity.	(+) Seniors participating in athletic events at an advanced age have often been engaged in physical activity throughout their lives; school physical education influences lifelong engagement in sports.
Myers and Hamilton (1985); 128 older adults, ages 55 to 101 (avg. age = 74.2). From 11 Fun and Fitness groups from 4 provinces sponsored by the Canadian Red Cross. Subjects from general community, seniors' apartments, institutional care. Studied over 12 to 48 months.	Survey of background; patterns of physical activity, perceived difficulty with activities of active daily living (ADL).	(+) Participants substantially increased their participation with time; program acted as motivator; program catered to inactive but healthy seniors. Once a week session may not result in physical improvement, thus participants must be aware of exercising outside of the program (i.e., more than once/week); majority of participants (58%) engaged in more than one activity.

Cross-sectional studies have found correlations among various lifestyle behaviors. For example, Leigh and Fries (1992–1993) found that exercise behavior was negatively correlated with smoking and positively correlated with high-fiber diet, being male, and being highly educated.

Alcoholism is a progressive, chronic disease that affects all aspects of an alcoholic's life — body, mind, and spirit (Palmer, Vaic, & Epstein, 1988). Compared to alcohol abuse among young and middle-aged adults, alcohol abuse among the elderly has received very little attention (e.g., Carstensen et al., 1985). Even less attention has been given to the effects, if any, of physical activity as a form of treatment program for alcoholism. Emphasis in the literature alludes to the social networking and support systems which physical activity provides in treatment, as well as the contribution to emotional health and general well-being. However, more systematic research is needed.

Discussion of the Evidence

Smoking is the risk factor most commonly studied for its correlation with exercise, but few studies have included older (or middle age) adults. Some research has found a negative correlation between physical activity and smoking, suggesting that smoking is associated with less activity (Marti et al., 1988; Salonen et al., 1991; cited in Wankel & Sefton, 1993). Both of those studies included 30- to 59-year-olds of both sexes.

Rehm et al. (1993) examined the effects of alcohol consumption, smoking, physical activity, and close personal relationships on mortality. There were 1,668 subjects in a longitudinal study over 13 years. While alcohol intake and smoking elevated the mortality rate, physical activity and the availability of a steady partner had protective effects. However, the interrelationship of alcohol use and activity was not clear. Other studies which do support an activity/alcohol use relationship were conducted on adults younger than age 50 (Gary & Guthrie, 1972; Palmer, Vace, and Epstein, 1988).

The potential role of physical fitness in recovery from all forms of uncontrolled dependence is an important factor in the design of effective recovery programs. Fridinger and Dehart (1993) suggested that alcohol and other substance abuse treatment programs are now focusing more on the total patient rather than just targeting functional sobriety. They also provided a model for a suggested treatment program utilizing physical conditioning and healthful nutritional habits to improve the chances of recovery.

The interrelationship among lifestyle behaviors of older adults needs a lot more study. Most research has focused on the relationship of each individual lifestyle behavior to morbidity and/or mortality, usually controlling for the influence of other risk factors. How the behaviors themselves cluster has been of less interest to researchers.

MEDICATION USE OUTCOMES

The level of evidence for the influence of physical activity on medication use outcomes is **weak**. There is little research on this issue, although on occasion medication use is included as a variable in studies focusing on other health outcomes. For example, Allegrante et al. (1993) found that medication use was decreased at a level approaching statistical significance in a group of arthritis patients compared to controls in a walking program.

There are significant problems underlying the study of medication use and physical activity. For example, a huge variety of medications exist for varying conditions, and each has a specific function. Physical activity may effect certain aspects of medication use, but the specificity of each type of medication makes research difficult. Furthermore, older adults often take combinations of medications, and there are individual differences in reactions. Finding adequate sample sizes to discover associations is a challenge.

The National Advisory Council on Aging (1994) suggested that 25 percent to 40 percent of all prescriptions consumed are inappropriate, and that 15 percent of hospital admissions are a result of drug reactions. Drug expenditures represented the largest rise in health care costs between 1987 and 1991, and they rank third in total expenditures behind hospital use and physician services. Seniors, the largest group of medication consumers, comprise 12 percent of the population, yet consume 25 percent of prescribed medications. If physical activity could play a role in reducing older adults' medication needs, there would be cost savings for individuals (both monetary and reduced drug dependency) and for the health care system.

STRESS AND COPING OUTCOMES

Summary

The level of evidence for a relationship between physical activity and stress and coping among older adults is **weak**. Very few studies have investigated the relationship between a physically active lifestyle and older adults' experience of and ability to cope with stressful life events or chronic stressors.

There are some indications that exercise may moderate the psychological and somatic effects of stress for the elderly. However, future studies need to look specifically at the conditions under which this moderation would occur. Future research needs to examine different types of stressors (e.g., chronic stressors like loneliness or low income, versus stressful events like moving to a nursing home or death of a spouse) as well as between different types of effects (physical, psychological, behavioral).

Discussion of the Evidence

While some studies have investigated this relationship for middle-aged adults (e.g., Blumenthal et al., 1991; Howard et al, 1984; Roskies et al., 1986), research in this area among the elderly is scant. One correlational study (Speake et al., 1991) compared elderly from urban areas with those living in rural areas and found no significant differences on a stress management measure between the two groups. However, the physical activity levels of these groups were only assumed, not measured.

Two studies have looked at the effects of an exercise intervention program on the perceived amount of stress experienced by younger elderly (mean age around 57 years). Of these two, King et al.'s (1993) involved the largest sample and the longest program. The results of this study suggested that regular exercise may indeed reduce the amount of stress experienced, but more so among elderly who exercise at home than among those who exercise in a group outside their home. The other study (Norvell et al., 1991) did not find significant differences between exercisers and nonexercisers after a 12-week program; however, there was an inverse relationship between aerobic capacity and amount of stress perceived.

Various theoretical perspectives predict a positive effect of physical activity on the experience of and reaction to stress. It has been proposed, for instance, that physical activity may moderate the experience of stress by

(a) providing social support,
(b) providing an effective outlet for repressed anger and frustration or
(c) substituting the ambiguous stresses of daily living with a concrete, specific physiological stress. Furthermore, it has been suggested that fit individuals are better able to recover from an induced state of sympathetic arousal.

Although a moderating effect of physical activity on reactions to stress has been corroborated for younger age groups (Howard et al., 1984), it is far from clear to what extent and under which conditions this relationship may hold for elderly people. For example, King et al.'s study suggested that social contact through physical activity may not play a role in the activity-stress relationship among the elderly, as it may in younger age groups (Howard et al., 1984).

In conclusion, more research is necessary to clarify the relationship between physical activity and stress among the elderly. Future studies need to look specifically at the parameters of the physical activity-stress relationship: under what conditions might exercise have a buffering effect on the experience of and reaction to stress, as well as the types of reactions to stress (physiological, psychological, behavioral)? Table 5-3 presents intervention/comparison studies; no physical activity-specific correlational/epidemiological studies were reviewed.

ACTIVITIES OF DAILY LIVING (FUNCTIONAL INDEPENDENCE) OUTCOMES

Summary

The level of evidence for a relationship between physical activity and the degree to which older adults can carry out activities of daily living (ADLs) is **suggestive** and consistent, though more prospective intervention studies are needed to clarify the specific benefits of an active lifestyle in promoting functional independence.

ADLs and instrumental activities of daily living (IADLs) refer to self-maintenance activities that are reflective of mobility or physical functioning (e.g., Katz, 1983). ADLs include such basic activities as eating, dressing, bathing, or moving around (e.g., sitting and standing). IADLs include intermediate-level activities such as housekeeping, shopping, and transportation. More recently, researchers have examined advanced activities of daily living (AADLs; Reuben et al., 1990), which are voluntary activities such as travelling, hobbies, recreational exercise, employment, and participation in social and religious groups.

Most of the research presented in Tables 5-4 and 5-5 has examined basic ADLs. Physical activity is positively correlated with ADLs in both cross-sectional and prospective studies, and various exercise interventions have been shown to improve and/or maintain functioning in basic ADLs. The results obtained were consistent across correlational and intervention studies for different measures of ADLs (e.g., tiredness, dependence on help from others), and for different types of physical activity (e.g., walking, gardening, aerobic exercises, strength exercises, seated exercises). Some research (e.g., Avlund et al., 1994) found a dose-response relationship between intensity of physical activity (light vs. heavy) and ADLs.

Women and men both seem to benefit from physical activity. Although men scored higher on a number of the exercise measures (in absolute terms) in most of the studies, there were no differences in the relationship of exercise with ADLs.

Table 5-3
Stress and Coping Outcomes: Intervention and Comparison Studies

Researchers and sample	Design, treatment, and measures	Findings
King et al. (1993); 357 older adults (160 F, 197 M), ages 50 to 65 (avg. age = 56.2 M, 57.0 F). From private residences of Sunnyvale, CA; recruited through random telephone survey. No heart disease or stroke; no physical activity program for last 6 months.	Subjects randomly assigned to groups. High-intensity–group-based exercise (HG): 60 min of which 40 min walk/jog; 3 times/week, up to 73% to 88% of max HR. High-intensity–home-based exercise (HH): 60 min of which 40 min walk/jog, 3 times/week; up to 73% to 88% of max HR. Low-intensity–home-based (LH): 30 min brisk walking, 5 times per week, 60% to 73%. Assessment only control (C). 12 months for all groups. 16% dropout after 1 year; greater adherence for HH and LH (75%) than for HG. Measures: VO_2 max treadmill; Perceived Stress Scale (PSS); ratings of perceived change in experienced stress.	(+) Significantly lower PSS stress scores post-program for HH and LH than for controls; HH and LH decreased over time. Significant improvement in perceived changes in stress in exercisers vs. control; no significant differences among HG, HH, & LH. Significant improvement in VO_2 max and treadmill for HG, HH, and LH, not controls.
Norvell et al. (1991); 43 F; avg. age = 58.9; sedentary, postmenopausal.	Random assignment to one of three groups: Aerobic: 30 min cycle ergometer; 2 times per week for 12 weeks at 70% to 85% of max HR. Passive: exercise tables. Controls: no exercise. Measures: VO_2 max bicycle test, weight, skinfold, girth. Perceived Stress Scale.	(−) No significant improvement on Perceived Stress Scale for any of the groups. (+) Significant improvement in VO_2 max for aerobic group; improvement in VO_2 max was positively correlated with changes in PSS scores.

Table 5-4
Activities of Daily Living Outcomes: Intervention and Comparison Studies

Researchers and sample	Design, treatment, and measures	Findings
O'Hagan et al. (1994); 71 subjects (sex not specified); avg. age = 83 in exercise group (range 62 to 102); 80 in control group (range 62 to 95). Frail elderly; 11 residential homes; Three homes chosen for exercise classes, eight for controls (subjects randomly selected from these). Volunteer subjects (none excluded for medical reasons).	Two groups: 34 subjects in exercise group: Full range of motion, strength, coordination, flexibility and balance. Warm-up, aerobic activity, cool-down. Weekly one-hour and twice weekly ten-min exercise classes. Set to old-time music and supervised by a P.T. Control group (37 subjects): regular residential activities. 12-month program. 64.7% of exercise group and 62.1% of control group completed the study. Measures: sit stand test at 4, 9, and 12 months. Assessed time taken to stand up, level of hand assistance.	(+) No baseline differences between groups. No change in control group over the 12 months. Exercise group improved in first four months and maintained improvement for rest of 12-month period. Most of exercise group also maintained their daily level of physical activity, whereas half of control group declined.
McMurdo and Rennie (1993); 49 older adults (33F, 8M), avg. age = 81 (range 63 to 91). From four residential homes in Dundee, Scotland; residents invited to volunteer for study. Only those with severe communication difficulties excluded. Many frail.	Nonrandom assignment to one of two groups. 15 subjects in exercise group: 7 months of seated exercises, 10 min warm-up, 35 min exercise to put upper and lower limb joints through full range of motion; mostly strength exercises. Reminiscence group (26 subjects): 7 months; music and reminiscence (45 min) to promote social inter-action. Twice per week for both groups. Attrition: 33% from exer-cise, 11.5% from reminiscence. Avg. attendance 91% for exercise, 86% for reminiscence. ADL meas-ures: Barthel Index; spinal flexion by bending with knees straight and reaching toward floor; chair-to-stand by rising from straight-backed chair without using hands.	(+) Exercise groups improved on all functional measures; reminiscence group deteriorated.

(Continued)

Table 5-4

(*Continued*)

Researchers and sample	Design, treatment, and measures	Findings
Sulman and Wilkinson (1989); 20 older adults (9F, 11M), all over 70. 8 examined for 6-month time period (1 F, 7 M); 3 more women followed for 3 months. Canadian hospital patients in a long-stay activity program. No control group.	Subjects did seated exercises such as arm and leg raises, joint rotations, beach ball toss, plastic horseshoes and other tossing activities. 45 min sessions, 5 days per week. 40% of original 20 participated for six months out of a possible 10. Ten patients enrolled in group at any given time, but avg. six patients attended each session. Measures: Trimodal Ability Profile (regular daily activities like eating and dressing); London Psychogeriatric Rating Scale (included physical disability scale); physical skills in the group program also rated. Scales used on nursing unit; staff ratings in program (run by O.T.s and social workers).	(+) In general, study patients either improved or maintained function. Six of eight improved in functioning on group activities, other two maintained; three of eight patients improved ADLs, two maintained.

This suggests that the important issue is exercise has benefits relative to one's own capabilities.

Discussion of the Evidence

LaCroix et al. (1993) suggested several reasons for the positive relationship between physical activity and the maintenance of mobility and independent living in later life. Increased bone density; improved lipid profiles; increased strength, balance, and coordination; improved aerobic capacity; and decreased depression are likely to translate to reduced risks of coronary events, osteoporotic fractures, and mortality. LaCroix et al. (1993) also suggested that the benefits of physical activity not only prevent chronic diseases, but also reduce frailty. They defined frailty as "an increased susceptibility to disability resulting from diminished physiologic reserve" (p. 867). LaCroix et al. (1993) examined a number of lifestyle behaviors in their study, and concluded that physical activity appears to have the greatest po-

Table 5-5

Activities of Daily Living Outcomes: Correlational and Epidemiological Studies

Researchers and sample	Measures	Findings
Avlund et al. (1994); 541 older adults surveyed, 405 provided complete data (196 F, 209 M). All ages 75. Random sample from 11 Danish municipalities. Cross-sectional; one point in time.	Survey question about physical activity (six possible levels, ranging from "hardly any" to "hard or very hard exercise regularly." Functional ability scale developed for study. Subjects indicated whether they could do activities related to mobility and upper/lower limb function "with or without being tired afterwards" or "with or without help." Activity items combined to reflect three "tiredness" scales and two "dependence" (help) scales (the latter combined upper and lower limb function into a single ADL score). Subjects also did walking test (speed over 10m; 1.4 m/s was cutoff for high and low physical functioning). Step test (highest step achieved without assistance from handrail; 40 cm criterion).	(+) Regular and more vigorous exercise was significantly related to less tiredness and higher independence scores. Poor performance in step tests associated with dependence in both mobility and ADL for men; tiredness in mobility for women. Limitations in walking tests associated with greater tiredness in mobility function for both women and men; and dependence in mobility function in women (more than 11 times increase in odds ratio in this analysis).

(*Continued*)

Table 5-5
(*Continued*)

Researchers and sample	Measures	Findings
Kaplan et al. (1993); 580 older adults; 508 completed 1984 interviews; 356 completed 1990 interviews (209 F, 147 M), ages 65 or older. Over-65 (in 1984) were a subset of the Alameda County (CA) study.	5-item exercise scale: takes part in sports, walks for exercise, exercises long enough to work up a sweat, does calisthenics or stretches, does any other vigorous exercise. Scale developed for survey included: activities of daily living (ADLs), such as bathing and dressing; instrumental activities of daily living (IADLs) such as cooking and shopping, physical mobility items such as walking a half mile and climbing a flight of stairs; physical performance items such as lifting a 10-lb weight or moving objects; getting around to places person wants to go.	(+) Active older adults maintain physical function better than less active older adults. Baseline exercise score was positively associated with overall change in functional ability score from 1984–1990. Relationship of exercise score to specific types of functional ability were not reported.
LaCroix et al. (1993); 6,981 older adults (3,935 F, 3,046 M); ages 65 and over. Taken from Established Populations for Epidemiologic Studies of the Elderly. Random community samples from Massachusetts, Iowa, and Connecticut. 4-year study.	Self-reported frequency of walks, gardening, and vigorous exercise. Classified as frequently (3 or more times per week); sometimes (at least once per week); rarely, or never. Self-reported ability to walk a half mile or walk up and down stairs.	(+) Those who frequently were active were most likely to maintain mobility; those who never engaged in activity were least likely to maintain mobility. Different types of exercise showed similar results.

(*Continued*)

Table 5-5

(Continued)

Researchers and sample	Measures	Findings
Borchelt and Steinhagen-Thiessen (1992); 450 older adults (207 F, 243 M). Old: ages 70 to 84 (212 subjects), avg. age 77.4. Very old (238 subjects), avg. age 92. Random sample of adults ages 70 to 105 living in private households and institutions in West Berlin. From residential registry, stratified by age-sex. Cross-sectional.	Physical vigor measured by dynamometer grip strength; self-reported maximum walking distance. Katz Index for ADL.	(+) Walking distance was a significant predictor of ADL. No gender differences in this prediction, though males as a group scored higher than females as a group on both walking and grip strength.
Duffy and McDonald (1990); 179 older adults (98 F, 69 M), avg. age = 74.1. Purposive sample through staff who manage various seniors' organizations. Mostly Caucasian with high school education or less. Cross-sectional.	Health Promoting Lifestyle Profile (included physical activity subscale). OARS Multi-dimensional Functional Assessment Questionnaire (incl. ADL subscale).	(+) Exercise subscale positively correlated with OARS (correlation with ADL subscale not reported). Age subgroup analyses showed younger old (65 to 74) to have highest ADL but lowest exercise scores; oldest old (85+) had highest exercise but lowest ADL.

tential for reducing susceptibility to mobility losses. They recommended adapting physical activities to a broad range of capabilities and health concerns to facilitate exercise participation in older adults.

One finding among the research reviewed here seems puzzling. Duffy and McDonald (1990) found that adults over 85 had the lowest ADL scores but the highest self-reported exercise; whereas those ages 65 to 74 had the highest ADL but lowest exercise scores. It is possible that the old-old engaged in exercise to prevent further deterioration in mobility, while the young-old did not perceive themselves as vulnerable to mobility loss so they did not feel the need to exercise for reasons of prevention. Alternatively, the frail state of the old-old may have led them to overestimate their exercise participation. These issues await further study.

Most of the correlational studies have been cross-sectional. More prospective and intervention studies are needed. Conclusions from cross-sectional research are limited because restricted mobility could be the cause, rather than the effect, of restricted physical activity (e.g., Borchelt & Steinhagen-Thiessen, 1992). The intervention research to date has (a) relied on small samples, (b) not focused on age differences and wide ranges of ability/disability, and (c) been restricted to institutional settings. It would be of particular interest to study the role of physical activity in preventing or delaying institutionalization by improving or maintaining functioning.

Less work has been done on the relationship between physical activity and intermediate or advanced ADLs than on basic ADLs. Deterioration of function with respect to IADLs or AADLs is often a precursor to loss of ability to perform basic ADLs (e.g., Reuben et al., 1990), so the potential of exercise to maintain higher levels of function is an important question for further research.

Research on AADLs can also shed light on the potential of physical activity for enhancing social networks and activities and related social support. These variables are usually studied by exercise and health researchers as predictors rather than outcomes of activity involvement. However, AADLs (which include a number of social activities) can be studied as outcomes of physical activity. For example, Reuben et al. (1990) found that level of exercise was related to frequency of travel among elderly subjects, but not to local visiting in each others' homes. The implication was that an active lifestyle could lead to broader social networks and permit longer-range travel.

Stewart and King (1991) reviewed the impact of exercise on various quality of life outcomes. Emery and Blumenthal (1990) found that older adult participants in either an aerobic or yoga class (16 weeks) perceived that their social life was improved, relative to a control group. Stewart and King suggested that physical activity can enhance older adults' ability to function in social activities by improving physical functioning and mobility, and that participation can also provide friendship opportunities. In a study of retirees from the Campbell's Soup Company, Rudman (1987) found that retirees gave social contact as a reason for participating in a company-sponsored exercise program. More recently, O'Brien Cousins (1995) found that current exercise level was related to perceived social support in a sample of 327 elderly women in Vancouver. She suggested that such perceived social support and enhanced social networks in turn encourage maintenance of physical activity.

Chapter 6

Economic Outcomes

ECONOMIC OUTCOMES

Summary

The level of direct evidence for economic benefits of physical activity among older adults is **weak**. More is known about indirect economic outcomes such as extending healthy life span, curbing degree of illness during the life span, and fostering independent living; these are cost-effective to society and enhance quality of life for the individuals involved. Keeler et al. (1989) suggested that those who lead more sedentary lives cost society more through reduced work productivity, increased health care utilization, and high requirements for personalized care as they age. Shephard (1987) suggested that exercise programs can reduce the need for costly institutional care by increasing the physical capacity of sedentary adults to that of adults 10 to 20 years younger.

Physical activity may also prevent further deterioration and moderate symptoms among older adults who have developed disabilities (Schroll, 1994), thus having an economic impact through preventing of dependency and disability in later life stages. The implication of increased functional ability suggests personal independence and improved quality of life for older adults, therefore postponing or removing the likelihood of institutionalization. However, some experts suggest that any savings or gains may be minimal. Longer living adults may still encounter chronic health problems in late life, even if active life expectancy is extended. Although per capita rates of arthritis and other disabling factors have shown reduction (U.S. Department of Health and Human Services [USDHHS], 1994), Guralnik et al.'s (1991) three-year study of an elderly population found that disability but not disease rates are increasing with increasing age. It should be made clear that support services, more than acute health care, will require more funding than in the past.

The economic benefits of physical activity for the elderly are an important issue for government health care policy, given the aging population. In Canada and the United States, the elderly are the fastest-growing segment of the population. In 1991, there were 3.2 million Canadians over age 65; the proportion of seniors in the general population grew from 10 percent in 1981 to 12 percent in 1991 (Government of Canada, 1994[1]). The proportion of seniors 75 and over grew by 22 percent from 1981 to 1991 and the proportion of seniors 85 and over increased by 31 percent over the same 10-year period. There are currently about 100,000 Canadians and one million Americans over age 90.

According to the National Advisory Council on Aging (1994), older adults are the largest consumers of health care expenditures. Comprising 12 percent of the population, seniors use 25 percent of prescription medications, visit doctors more frequently, and have longer hospital stays than other age groups. Canadian seniors already account for 40 percent of all health care expenditures, an estimated $24 billion in 1990. In Ontario, where older adults (65 and over) account for only 10 percent of the population, they use 44 percent of beds in acute care hospitals.

Discussion of the Evidence

To date, few studies have focused on the economic benefits (to society and/or individuals) of physical activity among the elderly. Shephard (1993) suggested that exercise plays an important preventive role in many of the situations which lead to institutionalization, including acute medical crises, loss of social support, and functional loss. In addition, data from the Canada Health Survey (Health & Welfare Canada, 1983) indicate that the typical sedentary person faces about 10 years of partial dependency and a final year of total dependency. Active individuals are likely to be less reliant on institutional support as a lower proportion of exercisers require support at any given age compared with nonexercisers (Taylor, 1992). Shephard (1993) pointed out that exercise does not appear to extend longevity much beyond age 80; only a small proportion of exercisers survive to the point that institutional support is required.

One study conducted by the Department of Medicine at Stanford University (Lane et al., 1987) involved 498 long distance runners ages 50 to 72 years and 365 community controls. The researchers examined associations of repetitive, long-term physical impact (running) with musculoskeletal disability and medical service utilization over a number of years. They found that less money was

---

[1]Government of Canada. (1994). *Seniors in Canada: A decade in review.* Ottawa: National Advisory Council on Aging.

spent by runners on health care services than controls. Runners had significantly less physician visits per year (2.1 to 2.6), and about 30 percent of runners' visits were for running-related injuries. In addition, runners used fewer medications than did control subjects (0.52 versus 1.1). In other words, runnners' health care costs were lower both for the runners themselves and for society at large.

Leigh and Fries (1992) studied 1,558 former Bank of America employees (average age 69) for 12 months. In the one-year period of the study, relationships between health habits and subsequent medical costs were analyzed. Although the more active people had significantly lower health care costs, Leigh and Fries also noted that people who exercised 100 or more minutes per week paid an average of $50 to $362 per year for athletic equipment and fees, so overall cost savings were not clear.

In a study by Hatziandreu et al. (1988), cost-effectiveness analysis was used to estimate the health and economic implications of exercise in preventing coronary heart disease (CHD). Based on their estimates and assumptions, they concluded that exercise was a cost-effective approach to lowering the risk of CHD. Exercise cost $11,313 per Quality Adjusted Life Years (QALY) saved. These figures compare favorably with other published cost-effectiveness studies of CHD interventions (Paffenbarger et al., 1984). This cost-effectiveness analysis also provided calculations and analysis of time trade-off. Hatziandreu et al. (1988) estimated that the 1,000 men age 35 who exercised three times per week for 20 minutes for the next 30 years would spend a total of 522.7 years (as a group) in exercise, whereas 530 years would be gained by preventing CHD. The "benefit-cost" difference was positive by 7.3 years, representing a net gain of 2.7 days per member of the cohort.

Economic impact also needs to be examined in the area of falls prevention. Costs associated with fractures, injury, and surgery resulting from falls in the elderly may be moderated with physical activity. More work needs to carried out to determine to what degree balance can be improved, and how better balance may be related to falls prevention. The argument that physically active elderly are more at risk of falls simply because they are mobile needs scientific clarification; health benefits of activity have to be compared to the risks.

There is very little direct investigation regarding economic impact and more general active living outcomes. The challenge of assessing the economic impact of the more general concept of "active living" may be even greater than the challenge has been in assessing the health outcomes of the more specifically defined "vigorous physical activity," given the difficulties in operationalizing "active living." Moreover, researchers are just beginning to appreciate the complexity of gender, age, and social structure in determining leisure choices, physical activity patterns, health outcomes, and health care utilization. Moreover some of the benefits found may have large social value but no direct economic value in terms of cost savings. There is an ethical issue in focusing on individuals as economic units that either save or cost the health care system money. Economic outcomes of physical activity need to be considered in conjunction with social and other "quality of life" outcomes for individuals and communities. From a policy perspective, health promotion through increased physical activity makes ethical and economic sense. Promoting healthy aging has the potential to reduce unnecessary suffering from preventable illness.

Some researchers and practitioners have suggested using financial incentives tied to life insurance or taxation to encourage exercise. It is unclear whether such strategies would induce enough additional physical activity among sedentary, elderly adults to justify the costs (Keeler et al., 1989). Also, suggestions to reward healthy lifestyle behavior are somewhat controversial because health status is influenced by other factors besides lifestyle (e.g., genetic predisposition and socioeconomic status).

Innovative prospective and retrospective studies comparing active versus sedentary living over the life span for the timing, type, severity, and costs of disease onset, may ultimately illuminate the economic outcomes of physical activity participation. Such research may combine self-report with medical records of chronic diseases and disabilities (and associated costs).

Chapter 7

Limitations of Current Knowledge

SCIENTIFIC METHOD ADVANCES, LIMITS ACTIVE LIVING KNOWLEDGE

Current knowledge on active living outcomes among older adults is both advanced and limited by the scientific method. The more experimentally controlled the research design, the less the intervention is representative of the uncontrolled real world (see Chodzko-Zajko, 1994 for a thoughtful review of research designs with physical activity and older adults). In this section, research issues limiting our knowledge about older adults and the assessment of physical activity are presented.

The Definition of Active Living and Methods of Activity Assessment

While sport scientists acknowledge that exercise programs "do no harm," the empirical evidence supporting this claim is incomplete. One reason is that experimental studies use exercise interventions which are highly controlled, medically supervised, and biased (in terms of samples) toward healthy and more highly educated individuals. Thus the outcomes of these studies do not necessarily reflect the older adult activity experience either at home or in everyday programs as they occur in communities. Therefore, a broader perspective of physical activity, as reflected in the concept "active living," has not been well researched.

Even though this project review has encompassed over 1,500 scientific articles on physical activity, exercise, and sport, we still know little about how informal forms of daily activity affect older people's life quality and health. Some evidence exists to suggest that older people do place themselves at risk of falls and injuries in their daily activities around the home; evidence in controlled research settings also suggests that musculoskeletal injury is a realistic expectation for some elderly, especially in the early stages of undertaking a new activity and for those who take part in seriously competitive and high-challenge sport. However, many studies in this report illustrate the profound benefits that various levels of physical activity participation do have for older adults. Indeed, reversals in health and fitness are possible, and it must be acknowledged that simply slowing age declines should be considered to be a significant outcome.

Assessment of the activity levels and fitness of the elderly has shortcomings which add error and sampling bias. Often the assessments themselves are either too demanding or too crude to capture fitness or motor performance adequately. In the majority of studies, the physiological benefits of aerobic exercise are defined in scientific terms and frequently assessed as statistically significant improvement in oxygen uptake capacity as measured on a medically monitored treadmill using either submaximal or maximal protocols (making comparisons between studies difficult), or by bicycle ergometry. In bicycle ergometry, the aerobic power of elderly subjects may be limited by local muscle mechanisms rather than aerobic capacity. Also, many intervention studies are using self-reported radial or carotid pulse checks during the exercise sessions to estimate whether participants are exercising at the target intensity (Blumenthal et al., 1989), even though evidence indicates that older adults may not be very competent in the task of pulse monitoring.

Grip strength has been reported in several studies, but again the protocol varies. Also, the lack of standardization in assessing balance in the elderly along with the challenge of finding a relationship between postural balance and the prevalence of falls is a problem in current research (e.g., Berg et al., 1992; Fernie et al., 1982; Lichenstein et al., 1989). Moreover, little information is available on the contribution of specific types of exercise to the maintenance or even promotion of balance and other types of physical and functional health.

Other important benefits, such as expanded social networks or the personal views of the participating elderly are not assessed to understand the meaning or subjective value of the program in their lives. In-depth interviews and qualitative analysis would be useful in this regard.

Research Samples

A review of current exercise intervention research reveals that many studies have used self-selected, convenience, or recruited samples which are nonrepresentative of the general population. Thus the findings of those studies should not be generalized to the population at large. Samples in many cases are limited to small groups of individuals, as larger randomized-control studies on cross-sections of the general population are generally cost-prohibitive. Some studies report "no change" results from exercise, when the descriptive data suggested remarkable benefits in a sample too small for statistical significance. Evidence exists that some older adults are in a downward spiral that no intervention can stop; these failing adults' scores do moderate the overall health benefits that are evident among other subjects in the same study. Beyond sampling limitations, many researchers have not randomly assigned their subjects into treatment and control conditions. In addition, samples frequently include only Caucasian adults who are relatively well educated, middle- to upper-class, and highly motivated to participate. Thus we do not know if the treatment effects can be expected from the less advantaged and/or less motivated elderly. Females, especially the very old, and ethnic groups (both male and female), are poorly represented in the fitness and cardiovascular disease literature.

Medical Screening

Medical status interviews or self-administered questionnaires are typically conducted as screening devices. Research selection bias is added when certain individuals are eliminated from a study. For example, Seals et al. (1984a) used a maximal treadmill stress test to screen for cardiovascular disease while other researchers have used extensive exclusionary criteria for their research subjects, including history of myocardial infarction, stroke, evidence of CHD, uncontrolled diabetes, emphysema, and abnormal ECG (e.g., Blair et al., 1984). In the Canada Fitness Survey (1985), the majority (over 60%) of older adult participants were screened out of the aerobic step-test for reasons of possible health risk. Thus, this federal study did not provide findings that could be called normative.

By medically screening, researchers are reducing risk of negative reactions to exercise (and the associated ethical problems), but are also omitting segments of the very part of the population most suited to gain from more active living. Added to this type of research selection bias is that of the self-selection of volunteer subjects, who may be more likely to be (or believe themselves to be) in good health than those who do not volunteer.

Only disease impact studies have actively sought out individuals who are already afflicted with serious medical problems. More studies are encouraged on random samples of the older adult population regardless of health status, while taking appropriate cautions to design a range of exercise protocols that are within subjects' capabilities and do not put them at higher than usual risk.

Exercise Treatments

Treatment conditions are often not precisely specified, and when they are specified, the exercise protocols vary substantially in frequency, intensity, duration, and type of exercise across studies. Some studies last 12 weeks, others a year or longer. When exercise programs are directly compared, no attention is paid to matching these important training criteria.

Body composition and VO_2max are commonly measured as estimates of fitness and aerobic power, but far less data are available on muscular strength, muscular endurance, flexibility, or balance. Yet, as far as health, independence, and quality of life are concerned, the latter physical measures may be more important to assess. For example, strength and balance may have implications for mobility, quality of life, and related activities of daily living.

The potential of exercise programs to provide encouragement, enjoyment, social support networks, and sources of health promotion information have not been well explored. Many psychological variables (e.g., self-efficacy, beliefs, attitudes, perceived social support) have been studied primarily as predictors, rather than outcomes, of activity involvement.

It would also be useful to compare the benefits of different types of physical activities. Although walking programs (Gueldner & Spradley, 1988) and aquatics programs (Weinstein, 1986) are popular offerings for seniors in North American communities, and have been scientifically touted as beneficial to elderly participants, little attempt has been made to compare these two types of exercise to determine their unique or similar physiological, social, and psychological contributions. A few studies have provided support for aquatic exercise programs for those adults who have joint or obesity problems (e.g., Stevenson et al., 1988; Whitley & Schoene, 1987) while other studies have advocated land-based exercise programs (e.g., Cunningham et al., 1982; Myers & Hamilton, 1985). Few studies have been designed which directly compare land- versus water-based programs. Such research would need to match instructions, movement intensity, and duration of the interventions. However, we recognize that the relative benefits of different activities will be somewhat a matter of individual preference and skill levels, so any conclusions based on averages would need to be arrived at with caution.

The benefits of regular and moderate physical activity may extend to other issues which have not been considered promising for intervention research in the past. For example, the posture and standing height of kyphotic women (Dowager's hump deformity) may be at least partially correctable with simple physical exercise. Unpublished work on the postural outcomes of easy trunk strengthening exercise has demonstrated that osteoporotic women with obvious kyphosis of the spine were able to straighten up the back enough to increase their upright standing height by as much as two inches after participating in the program.

Adherence to Active Lifestyles

Adherence in older adult exercise programs is no worse than for younger adults, with a 50 percent adherence rate. Several studies report quite good adherence (60 percent to 90 percent) in exercise training (e.g., Blumenthal et al., 1989; Molloy et al., 1988; Posner et al., 1992). The question arises as to whether attendance at scientifically controlled exercise settings encourages or undermines adherence to a regular, self-directed program of activity. Research in progress suggests that even in lifelong active elderly, there are frequent disruptions in involvement. Thus over the life course of an active individual, re-establishing involvement may be more important to study than how to maintain a consistent pattern—that is, lifelong active adults may be better described as "persistent returners" and "re-entry opportunists" with regard to their ability to persistently overcome disruptions which inevitably occur at each life stage.

Some work has suggested that the athleticism of so few elderly is proof that aging decline is largely a socially reinforced learning phenomenon, and the limited involvement of older women in particular speaks to the influence of restrictive lifelong gender barriers combined with socialization processes. The life course activity status of older people, their cohort experiences, and relationships to present activity levels require further qualitative and quantitative research. Although the more physically active elderly have functional characteristics representative of inactive adults decades younger, it is unclear whether higher functional fitness is reflective of current or past activity patterns. Unfortunately, few qualitative life review studies or longitudinal quantitative studies are available to assist our understanding of active living patterns over the life course.

To better understand lifelong involvement and late-life adherence to physical activity, it will be important to ask questions about appropriate exercise prescription and about the type of exercise modalities best enjoyed and best suited to the needs of older adults. Perhaps the largest oversight in exercise gerontology is the lack of qualitative data from the older participants themselves. Little is known about the perceptions of elderly participants in terms of exertion levels, enjoyment factors, and situations which promote late-life exercise. We know little about the program capabilities and preferences (e.g., for types of music) of older adults. At best, all we can say is that older adults are so heterogeneous that a range of program offerings will be required, from chair exercises and gentle mobility, to ice skating, tap dancing, and gymnastics (O'Brien Cousins & Burgess, 1992). Qualitative studies using focus groups, biographical interviews, and oral surveys are needed to understand what older adults perceive are the positive and negative outcomes of exercise involvement for them, and the meaning of physical activity in their lives. We also need to know what incentives, if any, are likely to support participation.

CONCLUSION

The research evidence regarding the health outcomes of a physically active lifestyle suggests that older adults are reaping significant biological, social, and psychological benefits similar to their younger adult counterparts. Optimal fitness and well-being offers older people a protective edge in a number of important ways.

Activity may slow many forms of physical decline by up to 50 percent. As reviewed in the earlier chapters of this book, physical activity can protect against or enhance the management of many adverse conditions such as heart disease, some forms of cancer, respiratory conditions, arthritis, diabetes, osteoporosis, anxiety, and depression, though the levels of evidence for these outcomes vary. Physical activity also appears to enhance various cognitive and neurological functions of the brain, other psychological outcomes such as self-efficacy for further activity, and functional independence as assessed through activities of daily living. Again, levels of evidence vary. Other positive aspects of functioning such as better coping, encouragement, and socially supportive networks need more research.

More research is also needed into the potential of physical activity for earlier detection of disease processes, a more rapid recovery following a bout of serious illness, a more optimal functioning of the immune system, and a decreased need for medications. Compared to the health complications that we know occur with multiple and long-term medication use, physically active living may be the safer preferred alternative and may indeed be the "best medicine" to enhance quality and quantity of life (Jokl, 1985).

Although concerns about sudden death caused by over-exertion are unfounded because of the rarity of this type of event, in the more intense physical challenges, older men, more than women, are susceptible to some physical risk. Also, with sport and the more competitive aspects of physical activity, the social and psychological rewards may be very high for certain older individuals, but so too are the prospects for acute or chronic musculoskeletal injury. While self-paced and moderate forms of physical activity are known to be low-risk and health-promoting for low-fitness elderly, future research is needed to determine whether the benefits of intense sport and externally paced competitive activities are an adequate trade-off for the greater liabilities which face highly active adults in their older years.

This report has summarized a good deal of evidence indicating that the benefits of physically active lifestyles are definitely worth the time and trouble when participants experience good instruction, facilities, and expert evaluation of personal progress. It is not known whether these same benefits would be obtained with untrained exercise leaders, in less than ideal facilities, and with little or no evaluation of the program outcomes. Such quality control is not always available in small community programs. What are the benefits for everyday seniors in lay programs taught by lay instructors, and how do these benefits differ from tightly controlled research interventions? What are the basic requirements for a community program to be effective, and what are the appropriate standards for professional versus lay personnel?

The benefits of everyday recreational activities also require further study. For summer activities, which gardening activities contribute best to aerobic fitness? To flexibility? To strength? Since many older adults do not sweat, and are not able to find their pulse, how can we guide older people to monitor their level of intensity for both fitness and safety? What are the risks and benefits of older people exercising alone in their homes? How should exercise prescription differ for the aged?

A reality for northern-dwelling older adults is that stairs, sidewalks, and lanes and roads are icy during many months of the year. Some older people stay indoors for days and weeks at a time, unable or unwilling to risk a fall outdoors. This raises many questions. What can research offer us as insight into the best way to overcome the activity limitations of North American winters? What are the risks versus benefits of winter walking for older adults? How should older people avoid falls out of doors? How much safer is mall walking? How slowly can people walk and still reap physiological benefits? If they do fall, can older adults reduce injury by learning landing techniques to absorb forces over time and distance? Do ski poles work better than a cane for winter walking in safety?

These and a host of other questions are bound to become pressing to fitness researchers and practitioners as more older people set themselves the goal of increasing their personal physical activity. Given the changing demographics of industrialized countries toward an older population, scientific study of the benefits of active living for older adults is a timely issue.

References

A.L.C.C.O.A. (1995). Report to the Active Living Coordinating Centre for Older Adults. *Active living outcomes among older adults: A critical review of the health benefits and other outcomes*. Edmonton, AB: University of Alberta.

American Psychological Association (APA), (1994). Publication Manual of the American Psychological Association (4th ed.) Washington, DC: APA.

Aoyagi, Y., & Katsuta, S. (1990). Relationship between the starting age of training and physical fitness in old age. *Canadian Journal of Sport Science, 15* (1), 65–71.

Arfken, C. L., Lach, H. W., McGee, S., Birge, S. J., & Miller, J. P. (1994). Visual acuity, visual disabilities and falling in the elderly. *Journal of Aging & Health, 6,* 38–50.

Aronow, W. S., & Ahn, C. (1994). Correlation of serum lipids with the presence or absence of coronary artery disease in 1,793 men and women age > 62 years. *The American Journal of Cardiology, 73,* 702–703.

Aronow, W. S., Starling, L., Etienne, F., D'Alba, P., Edwards, M., Lee, N. H., & Parungao, R. F. (1986). Risk factors for coronary artery disease in persons older than 62 years in a long-term health care facility. *The American Journal of Cardiology, 57,* 518–520.

Astrand, P. O. (1986). Exercise physiology of the mature athlete. In J. R. Sutton & R. M. Brock (Eds.), *Sportsmedicine for the mature athlete* (pp. 3–13). Indianapolis, IN: Benchmark Press.

Astrand, P. O. (1992). "Why exercise?". *Medicine & Science in Sports, 24,* 153–162.

Atkins, C. J., Kaplan, R. M., Timms, R. M., Reinsch, S., & Lofback, K. (1984). Behavioral exercise programs in the management of chronic obstructive pulmonary disease. *Journal of Consulting & Clinical Psychology, 52,* 591–603.

Avlund, K., Schroll, M., Davidsen, M., Levborg, B., & Rantanen, T. (1994). Maximal isometric muscle strength and functional ability in daily activities among 75-year-old men and women. *Scandinavian Journal of Medicine, Science, & Sports, 4,* 32–40.

Babcock, M. A., Paterson, D. H., & Cunningham, D. A. (1994). Effects of aerobic endurance training on gas exchange kinetics of older men. *Medicine & Science in Sports, 26,* 447–452.

Ballard, J. E., McKeown, B. C., Graham, H. M., & Zinkgraf, S. A. (1990). The effect of high level physical activity (8.5 METS or greater) and estrogen replacement therapy upon bone mass in postmenopausal females, aged 50–68 years. *International Journal of Sports Medicine, 11,* 208–214.

Bandura, A. (1977). Self-efficacy: toward a unifying theory of behavioral change. *Psychological Review*, *84*, 191–215.

Barnard, R. J. (1991). Effects of life-style modification on serum lipids. *Archives of Internal Medicine*, *151*, 1389–1394.

Bashore, T. R. (1989). Age, physical fitness, and mental processing speed. *Annual Review of Gerontology & Geriatrics*, *9*, 120–144.

Bashore, T. R., Martinerie, J. M., Weiser, P. C., Greenspan, L. W., & Heffley, E. F. (1988). Preservation of mental processing speed in aerobically fit older men. *Psychophysiology*, *25*, 433–434.

Baulch, Y. S., Larson, P. J., Dodd, M. J., & Doetrich, C. (1992). The relationship of visual acuity, tactile sensitivity, and mobility of the upper extremities to proficient breast self-examination in women 65 and older. *Oncology Nursing Forum*, *19*, 1367–1372.

Bautch, J. C. (1993). Effects of low-intensity exercise program on functional ability in individuals with osteoarthritis of the knee. Poster presented at the Gerontological Society of America Annual Scientific Meeting, New Orleans, November.

Baylor, A. M., & Spirduso, W. W. (1988). Systematic aerobic exercise and components of reaction time in older women. *Journal of Gerontology: Psychological Sciences*, *43*, P121–126.

Beck, B., Modlin, T., Heithoff, K., & Shue, V. (1992). Exercise as an intervention for behavior problems. *Geriatric Nursing*, 273–275.

Becker, M. H. (1974). The health belief model and personal health behavior. *Health Education Monographs*, *2*, 324–508.

Belman, M. J., & Gaesser, G. A. (1991). Exercise training below and above the lactate threshold in the elderly. *Medicine & Science in Sports*, *23*(5), 562–568.

Belman, M. J., & Kendregan, B. A. (1981). Exercise training fails to increase skeletal muscle enzymes in patients with chronic obstructive pulmonary disease. *American Review of Respiratory Disease*, *123*, 256–261.

Berg, K. O., Maki, B. E., Williams, J. I., Holliday, P. J., & Wood-Dauphinee, S. L. (1992). Clinical and laboratory measures of postural balance in an elderly population. *Archives of Physical Medicine & Rehabilitation*, *73*, 1073–1080.

Bild, D. E., Fitzpatrick, A., Fried, L. P., Wong, N. D., Haan, M. N., Lyles, M., Bovill, E., Polak, J. F., & Schulz, R. (1993). Age-related trends in cardiovascular morbidity and physical functioning in the elderly: The Cardiovascular Health Study. *Journal of the American Geriatrics Society*, *41*, 1047–1056.

Binder, E. F., Brown, M., Craft, S., Schechtman, K. B., & Birge, S. J. (1994). Effects of a group exercise program on risk factors for falls in frail older adults. *Journal of Aging & Physical Activity*, *2*, 25–37.

Blair, S. N. (1984). How to assess exercise habits and physical fitness. In J. D. Matarazzo, S. M. Weiss, J. A. Herd, & N. E. Miller (Eds.), *Behavioral health: A handbook for health enhancement and disease prevention* (pp. 424–427). New York: John Wiley & Sons.

Blair, S. N. (1993). Evidence for success of exercise in weight loss and control. *Annals of Internal Medicine*, *119*, 702–706.

Blankfort-Doyle, W., Waxman, H., Coughey, K., Naso, F., Carner, E. A., & Fox, E. (1989). An exercise program for nursing home residents. In A. C. Ostrow (Ed.), *Aging and motor behavior* (pp. 201–216). Indianapolis, IN: Benchmark Press.

Block, J. E., Smith, R., Friedlander, A., & Genant, H. K. (1989). Preventing osteoporosis with exercise: A review with emphasis on methodology. *Medical Hypotheses*, *30*, 9–19.

Blumenthal, J., Federikson, M., Matthews, K., Kuhn, C., Schiebolk, S., German, D., Rifai, N., Steege, J., & Rodin, J. (1991). Stress reactivity and exercise training in premenopausal and postmenopausal women. *Health Psychology, 10*, 384–391.

Blumenthal, J. A., Emery, C. F., Madden, D. J., Coleman, R. E., Riddle, M. W., Schniebolk, S., Cobb, F. R., Sullivan, M. J., & Higginbotham, M. B. (1991). Effects of exercise training on cardiorespiratory function in men and women > 60 years of age. *The American Journal of Cardiology, 67*, 633–639.

Blumenthal, J. A., Emery, C. F., Madden, D. J., George, L. K., Coleman, R. E., Riddle, M. W., McKee, D. C., Reasoner, J., & Williams, R. S. (1989). Cardiovascular and behavioral effects of aerobic exercise training in healthy older men and women. *Journal of Gerontology: Medical Sciences, 44*(5), M147–157.

Blumenthal, J. A., Emery, C. F., Madden, D. J., Schniebolk, S., Walsh-Riddle, M., George, L. K., McKee, D. C., Higginbotham, M. B., Cobb, F. R., & Coleman, R. E. (1991). Long-term effects of exercise on psychological functioning in older men and women. *Journal of Gerontology: Psychological Sciences, 46*, P352–361.

Blumenthal, J. A., Schocken, D. D., Needels, T. L., & Hindle, P. (1982). Psychological and physiological effects of physical conditioning on the elderly. *Journal of Psychosomatic Research, 26*, 505–510.

Bokovoy, J. L., & Blair, S. N. (1994). Aging and exercise: A health perspective. *Journal of Aging & Physical Activity, 2*, 243–260.

Bonner, A., & O'Brien Cousins, S. (1996). Exercise and Alzheimer's disease: Benefits and barriers. *Activities, Adaptation and Aging, 20*(4), 21–34.

Borchelt, M. F., & Steinhagen-Thiessen, E. (1992). Physical performance and sensory functions as determinants of independence in activities of daily living in the old and the very old. *Physiopathological Processes of Aging, 673*, 350–361.

Bouchard, C. (1994). Physical activity, fitness and health: Overview of the consensus symposium. In H. A. Quinney, L. Gauvin, & A. E. Wall (Eds.), *Toward active living* (pp. 1–14). Champaign, IL: Human Kinetics.

Brill, P. A., Burkhalter, H. E., Kohrt, H. W., Blair, S. N., & Goodyear, N. N. (1989). The impact of previous athletism on exercise habits, physical fitness, and coronary heart disease risk factors in middle-aged men. *Research Quarterly, 60*, 209–215.

Brill, P. A., Kohl, H. W., & Blair, S. N. (1992). Anxiety, depression, physical fitness, and all-cause mortality in men. *Journal of Psychosomatic Research, 36*, 267–273.

Brooks, J. D. (1993). Exercise: It adds life to our years, so why don't more people do it? Poster presentation presented at the Gerontological Society of America Annual Scientific Meeting, New Orleans, November.

Brown, D. F., & Jackson, T. W. (1994). Diabetes: 'tight control' in a comprehensive treatment plan. *Geriatrics, 49*, 24–34.

Brown, M., & Holloszy, J. O. (1991). Effects of a low-intensity exercise program on selected physical performance characteristics of 60- to 71-year-olds. *Aging, 3*, 129–139.

Butterworth, D. E., Nieman, D. C., Perkins, R., Warren, B. J., & Dotson, R. G. (1993). Exercise training and nutrient intake in elderly women. *Journal of the American Dietetic Association, 93*, 653.

Caird, F. I., Andrews, G. R., & Kennedy, R. D. (1973). Effect of blood pressure in the elderly. *British Heart Journal, 35*(5), 527–530.

Canada Fitness Survey. (1985). Sixty-year-old Canadians: A health and fitness profile. *Highlights/Fait-saillants, 63*, 1.

Canada Fitness Survey. (1988). Blueprint for action: Older adults and a healthy, active lifestyle. Fitness Canada: Secretariat for Fitness in the Third Age, Ottawa.

Canadian Fitness & Lifestyle Research Institute. (CFLRI). (1994). Active living among older adults: A critical review of health benefits and outcomes. Unpublished report. Ottawa, ON: CFLRI.

Carroll, J. F., & Pollock, M. L. (1992). Rehabilitation and life-style modification in the elderly [review]. *Cardiovascular Clinics, 22,* 209–227.

Carroll, J. F., Pollock, M. L., Graves, J. E., Leggett, S. H., Spitler, D. L., & Lowenthal, D. T. (1992). Incidence of injury during moderate- and high-intensity walking training in the elderly. *Journal of Gerontology: Medical Sciences, 47*(3), M61–66.

Carstensen, L., Rychtarik, R., & Prue, D. (1985). Behavioral treatment for the geriatric alcohol abuser: A long-term follow-up study. *Addictive Behaviors, 10,* 307–311.

Casaburi, R., Patessio, P., Ioli, F., Zanaboni, S., Donner, C., & Wasserman, K. (1991). Reductions in exercise lactic acidosis and ventilation as a result of exercise training in patients with obstructive lung disease. *American Review of Respiratory Disease, 143,* 9–18.

Caspersen, C. J., Bloemberg, B. P., Saris, W. H., Merritt, R. K., & Kromhout, D. (1991). The prevalence of selected physical activities and their relation with coronary heart disease risk factors in elderly men: the Zutphen Study, 1985. *American Journal of Epidemiology, 133,* 1078–1092.

Castelli, W. P., Wislon, P. W., Levy, D., & Anderson, K. (1989). Cardiovascular risk factors in the elderly. *The American Journal of Cardiology, 63,* 12–19.

Cheng, S., Suominen, H., & Heikkinen, E. (1993). Bone mineral density in relation to anthropometric properties, physical activity and smoking in 75-year-old men and women. *Aging Clinics in Experimental Research, 5,* 55–62.

Chodzko-Zajko, W. J. (1994). Experimental design and research methodology in aging: Implications for research and clinical practice. *Journal of Aging & Physical Activity, 2,* 360–372.

Chodzko-Zajko, W. J., Schuler, P., Solomon, J., Heinl, B., & Ellis, N. R. (1992). The influence of physical fitness on automatic and effortful memory changes in aging. *International Journal of Aging & Human Development, 35,* 265–285.

Christensen, H., & MacKinnon, A. (1993). The association between mental, social and physical activity and cognitive performance in young and old subjects. *Age & Ageing, 22,* 175–182.

Clark, B. A., Wade, M. G., Massey, B. H., & Van Dyke, R. (1975). Response of institutionalized geriatric mental patients to a twelve-week program of regular physical activity. *Journal of Gerontology, 30,* 565–573.

Clarkson-Smith, L., & Hartley, A. A. (1989). Relationships between physical exercise and cognitive abilities in older adults. *Psychology & Aging, 4,* 183–189.

Clarkson-Smith, L., & Hartley, A. A. (1990). Structural equation models of relationships between exercise and cognitive abilities. *Psychology & Aging, 5,* 437–446.

Clemons, J. J., & Foret, C. (1994). The effect of eight weeks of moderated simulated stair stepping (Stairmaster 4000PT) on physical working capacity and static balance of elderly adults. *Research Quarterly* (March), A-100.

Cockburn, J., Smith, P. T., & Wade, D. T. (1990). Influence of cognitive function on social, domestic, and leisure activities of community-dwelling older people. *International Disability Studies, 12,* 169–172.

Coggan, A. R., Spina, R. J., Rogers, M. A., King, D. S., Brown, M., Nemeth, P. M., & Holloszy, J. O. (1990). Histochemical and enzymatic characteristics of skeletal muscle in master athletes. *Journal of Applied Physiology, 68,* 1896–1901.

Connell, B. R. (1993). Patterns of naturally occurring falls among frail nursing home residents. Poster presentation at the 46th Gerontological Society of America Annual Scientific Meetings, New Orleans, November.

Cress, M. E., Thomas, D. P., Johnson, J., Kasch, F. W., Cassens, R. G., Smith, E. L., & Agre, J. C. (1991). Effect of training on VO_2max, thigh strength, and muscle morphology in septuagenarian women. *Medicine & Science in Sports, 23,* 752–758.

Crilly, R. G., Willems, D. A., Trenholm, K. J., Hayes, K. C., & Delaquierre-Richardson, L. F. O. (1989). Effect of exercise on postural sway in the elderly. *Gerontology, 35,* 137–143.

Cunningham, D. A., Paterson, D. H., Himann, J. E., & Rechnitzer, P. A. (1993). Determinants of independence in the elderly. *Canadian Journal of Applied Physiology, 18,* 243–254.

Cunningham, D. A., Rechnitzer, P. A., Pearce, M. E., & Donner, A. P. (1982). Determinants of self-selected walking pace across ages 19 to 66. *Journal of Gerontology, 37,* 560–564.

Cwikel, J. (1992). Falls among elderly people living at home: Medical and social factors in a national sample. *Israel Journal of Medical Sciences, 28,* 446–453.

Danielson, M. E., Cauley, J. A., & Rohay, J. M. (1993). Physical activity and its association with plasma lipids and lipoproteins in elderly women. *Annals of Epidemiology, 3,* 351–357.

Darga, L. L., Lucas, C. P., Spafford, T. R., Schork, M. A., Illis, W. R., & Holden, N. (1989). Endurance training in middle-aged male physicians. *Physician and Sports Medicine, 17,* 85–88; 91; 94; 97–98; 101.

Degre, S., Sergysels, R., Messin, R., Vandermoten, P., Salhadin, P. Denolin, H., & DeCoster, A. (1974). Hemodynamic responses to physical training in patients with chronic lung disease. *American Review of Respiratory Disease, 110,* 395–402.

Del Rey, P. (1982). Physical activity as a deterrent to the aging process: overview of a motor learning study on older adults. *Psycho-physiology, 17,* 3–4.

De Vries, H. A., Brodowicz, G. R., Robertson, L. D., Svoboda, M. D., Schendel, J. S., Tichy, A. M., & Tichy, M. W. (1989). Estimating physical working capacity and training changes in the elderly at the fatigue threshold (PWC). *Ergonomics, 32,* 967–977.

Dexter, P. A. (1992). Joint exercises in elderly persons with symptomatic osteoarthritis of the hip or knee. *Arthritis Care & Research, 5,* 36–41.

Dill, D. B., Robinson, S., & Ross, J. C. (1966). A longitudinal study of 16 champion runners. *Journal of Applied Physiology, 21,* 1251–1255.

Drinkwater, B. L. (1994). 1994 C. H. McCloy Research Lecture: Does physical activity play a role in preventing osteoporosis? *Research Quarterly, 65,* 197–206.

Drummond, A. (1990). Leisure activity after stroke. *International Disability Studies, 12,* 157–160.

Duffy, M. E., & MacDonald, E. (1990). Determinants of functional health of older persons. *The Gerontologist, 30,* 503–509.

Duncan, P. W., Chandler, J., Studenski, S., Hughes, M., & Prescott, B. (1993). How do physiological components of balance affect mobility in elderly men? *Archives of Physical Medicine & Rehabilitation, 74,* 1343–1349.

Duncan, P. W., Weiner, D. K., Chandler, J., & Studenski, S. (1990). Functional reach: A new clinical measure of balance. *Journal of Gerontology: Medical Sciences, 45*(6), M192–M197.

Dupler, T. L., & Cortes, C. (1993). Effects of whole-body resistive training in the elderly. *Gerontology, 39,* 314–319.

Durak, E. (1989). Exercise for specific populations: Diabetes mellitus. *Sports Training, Medicine, and Rehabilitation,* 175–180.

D'Urso, M., & Logue, G. (1988). Competitive adapted sports for impaired older adults. *Therapeutic Recreation Journal, 22,* 56–64.

Dustman, R. E., Emmerson, R. Y., Ruhling, R. O., Shearer, D. E., Steinhaus, L. A., Johnson, S. C., Bonekat, H. W., & Shigeoka, J. W. (1990). Age and fitness effects on EEG, ERPs, visual sensitivity, and cognition. *Neurobiology of Aging, 11,* 193–200.

Dustman, R. E., Emmerson, R. Y., & Shearer, D. E. (1990). Aerobic fitness may contribute to CNS health: Electrophysiological, visual and neurocognitive evidence. *Journal of Neuropsychology Research, 4,* 241–254.

Dustman, R. E., Ruhling, R. O., Russell, E. M., Shearer, D. E., Bonekat, H. W., Shigeoka, J. W., Wood, J. S., & Bradford, D. C. (1984). Aerobic exercise training and improved neuropsychological function of older individuals. *Neurobiology of Aging, 5,* 35–42.

Eck, L. H., Hackett-Renner, C., & Klesges, L. M. (1992). Impact of diabetic status, dietary intake, physical activity, and smoking status on body mass index in NHANES II. *The American Journal of Clinical Nutrition, 56,* 329–333.

Ehsani, A. A., Ogawa, T., Miller, T. R., Spina, R. J., & Jilka, S. M. (1991). Exercise training improves left ventricular systolic function in older men. *Circulation, 83,* 96–103.

Ekoe, J. M. (1989). Overview of diabetes mellitus and exercise. *Medicine and Science in Sports and Exercise,* 353–355.

Emery, C. F. (1994). Effects of age on physiological and psychological functioning among COPD patients in an exercise program. *Journal of Aging & Health, 6,* 3–16.

Emery, C. F., & Blumenthal, J. A. (1991). Effects of physical exercise on psychological and cognitive functioning of older adults. *Annals of Behavioral Medicine, 13,* 99–107.

Emery, C. F., & Gatz, M. (1990). Psychological and cognitive effects of an exercise program for community-residing older adults. *The Gerontologist, 30,* 184–188.

Emrich, E. (1985). Soziale determinanten sportlicher altivitaeten im alter - versuch einer empirishcen analyse. (Social aspects determining sport activities for the aging - an empirical study and analysis.). *Sportunterricht, 34,* 341–346.

Emrich, E. (1989). Sport im alter - sozialogische und sozialpsychologische aspekte. (Sports and the elderly - sociological and socio-psychological aspects). *Zeitschrift fur Gerontologie, 22,* 101–105.

Era, P., Jokela, J., & Heikkinen, E. (1986). Reaction time and movement times in men of different ages: A population study. *Perceptual & Motor Skills, 63,* 111–130.

Era, P., Rantanen, T., Avlund, K., Gause-Nilsson, I., Heikkinen, E., Schroll, M., Steen, B., & Suominen, H. (1994). Maximal isometric muscle strength and anthropometry in 75-year-old men and women in three Nordic localities. *Scandinavian Journal of Medicine, Science, & Sports, 4,* 26–31.

Fernie, G. R., Gryfe, C. I., Holliday, P. J., & Llewellyn, A. (1982). The relationship of postural sway in standing to the incidence of falls in geriatric subjects. *Age & Ageing, 11,* 11–16.

Ferraz, M. B., Ciconelli, R. M., Araujo, P. M., Oliveira, L. M., & Atra, E. (1992). The effect of elbow flexion and time of assessment on the measurement of grip strength in rheumatoid arthritis. *Journal of Hand Surgery - American Volume, 17,* 1099–1103.

Ferrini, R., Edelstein, S., & Barrett-Connor, E. (1994). The association between health beliefs and health behaviour change in older adults. *Preventive Medicine, 23,* 1–5.

Fiatarone, M. A., & Evans, W. J. (1993). The etiology and reversibility of muscle function in the aged. *Journal of Gerontology, 48(Special issue),* 77–83.

Fiatarone, M. A., Marks, E. C., Ryan, N. D., Meredith, C. N., Lipsitz, L. A., & Evans, W. J. (1990). High-intensity strength training in nonagenarians: Effects on skeletal muscle. *Journal of the American Medical Association, 263,* 3029–3034.

Fiatarone, M. A., Morley, J. E., Bloom, E. T., Benton, D., Solomon, G. F., & Makinodan, T. (1989). The effect of exercise on natural killer cell activity in young and old subjects. *Journal of Gerontology: Medical Sciences, 44*(2), M37–45.

Fiatarone, M. A., O'Neill, E. F., Doyle, N., Clements, K. M., Roberts, S. B., Kehayias, J. J., Lipsitz, L. A., & Evans, W. J. (1993). The Boston, FICSIT study: The effects of resistance training and nutritional supplementation on physical frailty in the oldest old. *Journal of the American Geriatric Society, 41,* 333–337.

Fiatarone, M. A., O'Neill, E. F., Doyle Ryan, N., Clements, K. M., Solares, G. R., Nelson, M. E., Roberts, S. B., Kehayias, J. J., Lipsitz, L. A., & Evans, W. J. (1994). Exercise training and nutritional supplementation for physical frailty in very elderly people. *New England Journal of Medicine: June 23, 330,* 1769–1775.

Fitzgerald, J. T., Singleton, S. P., Neale, A. V., Prasad, A. S., & Hess, J. W. (1994). Activity levels, fitness status, exercise knowledge, and exercise beliefs among healthy, older African American and white women. *Journal of Aging & Health, 6,* 296–313.

Foster, V. L., Hume, G. J. E., Byrnes, W. C., Dickinson, A. L., & Chatfield, S. J. (1989). Endurance training for elderly women: Moderate vs low intensity. *Journal of Gerontology: Medical Sciences, 44*(6), M184–188.

Fridinger, F., & Dehart, B. (1993). A model for the inclusion of a physical fitness and health promotion component in a chemical abuse treatment program. *Journal of Alcohol and Drug Education, 23,* 215–222.

Friedman, R., & Tappen, R. M. (1991). The effect of planned walking on communication in Alzheimer's Disease. *Journal of the American Geriatric Society, 39,* 650–654.

Frontera, W. R., Meredith, C. N., O'Reilly, K. P., & Evans, W.m. J. (1990). Strength training and determinants of VO_2max in older men. *Journal of Applied Physiology, 68,* 329–333.

Fuller, J. J., & Winters, J. M. (1993). Assessment of 3-D joint contact load predictions during postural/stretching exercises in aged females. *Annals of Biomedical Engineering, 21,* 277–288.

Gardner, A. W., & Poehlman, E. T. (1993). Physical activity is a significant predictor of body density in women. *The American Journal of Clinical Nutrition, 57,* 8–14.

Gary, V., & Guthrie, D. (1972). The effect of jogging on physical fitness and self-concept in hospitalized alcoholics. *Quarterly Journal of Studies on Alcoholism, 43,* 380–385.

Gerhardsson, D., Verdier, M., Steineck, G., Hagman, U., Rieger, A., & Norell, S. E. (1990). Physical activity and colon cancer: A case-referent study in Stockholm. *International Journal of Cancer, 46,* 985–989.

Gorbien, M. J., Bishop, J., Beers, M. H., Norman, D., Osterwiel, D., & Rubenstein, L. Z. (1992). Iatrogenic illness in hospitalized elderly people. *Journal of the American Geriatric Society, 40*, 1031–1042.

Gottlieb, S. O., & Gerstenblith, G. (1988). Silent myocardial ischemia in the elderly: Current concepts. *Geriatrics, 43*(4), 29–34.

Govindasamy, D., Paterson, D. H., Poulin, M. J., & Cunningham, D. A. (1992). Cardiorespiratory adaptation with short-term training in older men. *European Journal of Applied Physiology, 65*, 203–208.

Graham, D. F., Graham, I., & MacLean, M. J. (1991). Going to the mall: a leisure activity of urban elderly people. *Canadian Journal on Aging, 19*(4), 345–358.

Green, J., McKenna, F., Redfern, E. J., & Chamberlain, M. A. (1993). Home exercises are as effective as outpatient hydrotherapy for osteoarthritis of the hip. *British Journal of Rheumatology, 32*, 812–815.

Green, H. S., & Patla, P. E. (1992). Maximal aerobic power: Neuromuscular and metabolic considerations. *Medicine & Science in Sports & Exercise, 24*(1), 38–46.

Greendale, G. A., Hirsch, S. H., & Hahn, T. J. (1993). The effect of a weighted vest on perceived health status and bone density in older persons. *Quality of Life Research, 2*, 141–152.

Gronningsaeter, H., Hytten, K., Skauli, G., Christensen, C. C., & Ursin, H. (1992). Improved health and coping by physical exercise or cognitive behavioral stress management training in a work environment. *Psychology & Health, 7*, 147–163.

Grove, K. A., & Londeree, B. R. (1992). Bone density in postmenopausal women: High impact vs. low impact exercise. *Medicine and Science in Sports and Exercise, 24*, 1190–1194.

Gueldner, S. H., & Spradley, J. (1988). Outdoor walking lowers fatigue. *Journal of Gerontological Nursing, 14*, 6–12.

Guralnik, J. M., LaCroix, A. Z., Branch, L. G., Kasl, S. V., & Wallace, R. B. (1991). Morbidity and disability in older persons in the years prior to death. *American Journal of Public Health, 81*, 443–447.

Gurwitz, J. H., Sanchez-Cross, M. T., & Matulis, J. (1994). The epidemiology of adverse and unexpected events in the long-term care setting. *Journal of the American Geriatric Society, 42*, 33–38.

Hagberg, J., Graves, J. E., & Limacher, M. (1989). Cardiovascular responses of 70–79-year-old men and women to exercise training. *Journal of Applied Physiology, 69*(5), 792–798.

Hall, K. D., Hayes, K. W., & Falconer, J. (1993). Differential strength decline in patients with osteoarthritis of the knee: Revision of a hypothesis. *Arthritis Care & Research, 6*, 89–94.

Hallinan, C. J., & Schuler, P. B. (1993). Body-shape perceptions of elderly women exercisers and nonexercisers. *Perceptual & Motor Skills, 77*, 451–456.

Hamdorf, P. A., Withers, R. T., Penhall, R. K., & Haslam, M. V. (1992). Physical training effects on the fitness and habitual activity patterns of elderly women. *Archives of Physical Medicine & Rehabilitation, 73*, 603–608.

Hamdorf, P. A., Withers, R. T., Penhall, R. K., & Plummer, J. L. (1993). A follow-up study on the effects of training on the fitness and habitual activity patterns of 60- to 70-year-old women. *Archives of Physical Medicine & Rehabilitation, 74*, 473–477.

Hampson, S. E., Glasgow, R. E., Zeiss, A. M., Birskovich, S. F., Foster, L., & Lines, L. (1993). Self-management of osteoarthritis. *Arthritis Care & Research, 6,* 17–22.

Haskell, W. L. (1984). Overview: Health benefits of exercise. In J. D. Matarazzo, S. M. Weiss, J. A. Herd, & N. E. Miller (Eds.), *Behavioral Health* (pp. 409–423). John Wiley & Sons.

Hassmen, P., Ceci, R., & Backman, L. (1992). Exercise for older women: A training method and its influences on physical and cognitive performance. *European Journal of Applied Physiology, 64,* 460–466.

Hatfield, B. D., Goldfarb, A. H., Sforzo, G. A., & Flynn, M. G. (1987). Serum beta-endorphin and affective responses to graded exercise in young and elderly men. *Journal of Gerontology, 42,* 429–431.

Hatori, M., Hasegawa, A., Adachi, H., Shinozaki, A., Hayashi, R., Okano, H., Minunuma, H., & Murata, K. (1993). The effects of walking at the anaerobic threshold level on vertebral bone loss in postmenopausal women. *Calcified Tissue International, 52,* 411–414.

Hatziandreu, E. I., Koplan, J. P., Weinstein, M. C., Caspersen, C. J., & Warner, K. I. (1988). A cost-effectiveness analysis of exercise as health promotion activity. *American Journal of Public Health, 78,* 1417–1421.

Hawkins, H. L., Kramer, A. F., & Capaldi, D. (1992). Aging, exercise, and attention. *Psychology & Aging, 7,* 643–653.

Hawkins, W. E., Duncan, D. F., & McDermott, R. J. (1988). A health assessment of older Americans: Some multidimensional measures. *Preventive Medicine, 17,* 344–356.

Health & Welfare Canada. (1988). *Health promotion survey: Technical report.* Ottawa: Minister of Supply and Services.

Heath, G. W., Hagberg, J., Ehsani, A. A., & Holloszy, J. W. (1981). A physiological comparison of young and older endurance athletes. *Journal of Applied Physiology, 31*(3), 634–640.

Hein, H. O., Suadicani, P., Sorensen, H., & Gyntelberg, F. (1994). Changes in physical activity level and risk of ischemic heart disease: A six-year follow-up in the Copenhagen male study. *Scandinavian Journal of Medicine, Science, & Sports, 4,* 57–64.

Heislein, D. M., Harris, B. A., & Jette, A. (1994). A strength training study for postmenopausal women: A pilot study. *Archives of Physical Medicine & Rehabilitation, 75,* 198–204.

Hill, R. D., Storandt, M., & Malley, M. (1993). The impact of long-term exercise training on psychological function in older adults. *Journal of Gerontology: Psychological Sciences, 48,* P12–17.

Hogan, P. I., & Santomier, J. P. (1984). Effect of mastering swim skills on older adults' self-efficacy. *Research Quarterly, 55,* 294–296.

Hopkins, D. R., Murrah, B., Hoeger, W. W. K., & Rhodes, R. C. (1990). Effect of low-impact aerobic dance on the functional fitness of elderly women. *The Gerontologist, 30,* 189–192.

Hossack, K. F., & Bruce, R. A. (1982). Maximal cardiac function in sedentary normal men and women: Comparison of age-related changes. *Journal of Applied Physiology, 53*(4), 799–804.

Howard, J. H., Cunningham, D. A., & Rechnitzer, P. A. (1984). Physical activity as a moderator of life events and somatic complaints: A longitudinal study. *Canadian Journal of Applied Sport Sciences, 9,* 194–200.

Howze, E. H., Smith, M., & DiGilio, D. A. (1989). Factors affecting the adoption of exercise behavior among sedentary older adults. *Health Education Research, 4*, 173–180.

Hu, M., & Woollacott, M. J. (1994). Multisensory training of standing balance in older adults: I. Postural stability and one-leg stance balance. *Journal of Gerontology: Medical Sciences, 49*(2), M52–M61.

Hu, M., & Woollacott, M. H. (1994). Multisensory training of standing balance in older adults: II. Kinematic and electromyographic postural responses. *Journal of Gerontology: Medical Sciences, 49*(2), M62–M71.

Hultsch, D. F., Hammer, M., & Small, B. J. (1993). Age differences in cognitive performance in later life: Relationships to self-reported health and activity life style. *Journal of Gerontology: Psychological Sciences, 48*(1), P1–11.

Inbar, O., Oren, A., Scheinowitz, M., Rotstein, A., Dlin, R., & Casaburi, R. (1994). Normal cardiopulmonary responses during incremental exercise in 20- to 70-yr-old men. *Medicine & Science in Sports, 26*, 538–546.

Iverson, B. D., Gossman, M. R., Shaddeau, S. A., & Turner, M. E. (1990). Balance performance, force production, and activity levels in noninstitutionalized men 60 to 90 years of age. *Physical Therapy, 70*, 348–355.

Jirovec, M. M. (1991). The impact of daily exercise on the mobility, balance and urine control of cognitively impaired nursing home residents. *International Journal of Nursing Studies, 28*, 145–151.

Johansson, G., & Jarnlo, G. B. (1991). Balance training in 70-year-old women. *Physiotherapy Theory & Practice, 7*, 121–125.

Jokl, E. (1985). Excerpt from keynote speed at the Physical Activity, Aging and Sport Conference in West Point, New York.

Jonsson, P. V., Lipsitz, L. A., Kelley, M., & Koestner, J. (1990). Hypotensive responses to common daily activities in institutionalized elderly: A potential risk for recurrent falls. *Archives of Internal Medicine, 150*, 1518–1524.

Judge, J. O., Lindsey, C., Underwood, M., & Winsemius, M. (1993a). Balance improvements in older women: Effects of exercise training. *Physical Therapy, 73*, 254–265.

Judge, J. O., Whipple, R., King, M., & Wolfson, L. (1993b). Balance and resistance training: Effects on dynamic balance. *Clinical Research, 41*, 116A.

Julius, S., Amery, A., Whitlock, L. S., & Conway, J. (1967). Influence of age on hemodynamic response to exercise. *Circulation, 36*(2), 222–230.

Kahn, S. E., Larson, V. G., Beard, J. C., Cain, K. C., Fellingham, G. W., Schwartz, R. S., Veith, R. C., Stratton, J. R., Cerqueira, M. D., & Abrass, I. B. (1990). Effect of exercise on insulin action, glucose tolerance, and insulin secretion in aging. *American Journal of Physiology, 258*, E937–943.

Kallinen, M., & Alen, M. (1994). Sports-related injuries in elderly men still active in sports. *British Journal of Sports Medicine, 28*, 52–55.

Kaplan, G. A., Seeman, T. E., Cohen, R. D., Knudsen, L. P., & Guralnik, J. (1987). Mortality among the elderly in the Alameda County Study: Behavioral and demographic risk factors. *American Journal of Public Health, 77*, 307–312.

Kaplan, G. A., Strawbridge, W. J., Camacho, T., & Cohen, R. D. (1993). Factors associated with change in physical functioning in the elderly: A six-year prospective study. *Journal of Aging & Health, 5*, 140–153.

Kasch, F. W., Boyer, J. L., VanCamp, S. P., Verity, L. S., & Wallace, J. P. (1990). The effect of physical activity and inactivity on aerobic power in older men (A longitudinal study). *The Physician & Sportsmedicine, 18*, 73–77, 80, 83.

Kasch, F. W., Wallace, J. P., Van Camp, S. P., & Verity, L. (1988). A longitudinal study of cardiovascular stability in active men aged 45 to 65 years. *The Physician & Sportsmedicine, 16,* 117–119.

Katz, S. D., Bleiberg, B., Wexler, J., Bhargava, K., Steinberg, J. J., & LeJempel, T. H. (1993). Lactate turnover at rest and during submaximal exercise in patients with heart failure. *Journal of Applied Physiology, 75,* 1974–1979.

Kavanagh, T., & Shephard, R. J. (1990). Can regular sports participation slow the aging process? Data on Masters' athletes. *The Physician & Sportsmedicine, 18,* 94–102.

Keeler, E. B., Manning, W. G., Newhouse, J. P., Sloss, E. M., & Wasserman, J. (1989). The external costs of a sedentary life-style. *American Journal of Public Health, 79,* 975–981.

Keim, R. J., Cook, M., & Martini, D. (1992). Balance rehabilitation therapy. *Laryngoscope, 102,* 1302–1307.

Kelly, J. R. (1987). How they play in Peoria: Models of adult leisure. In G. A. Fine (Ed.), *Meaningful play, playful meaning* (pp. 35–44). Champaign, IL. Association for the Anthropological Study of Play: Human Kinetics.

Kelly, J. R., Steinkamp, M. W., & Kelly, J. R. (1987). Later-life satisfaction: Does leisure contribute? *Leisure Sciences, 9,* 189–200.

Keyser, R. E., DeLaFuente, K., & McGee, J. (1993). Arm and leg cycle cross-training effect on anaerobic threshold and heart rate in patients with coronary heart disease. *Archives of Physical Medicine & Rehabilitation, 74,* 276–280.

King, A. C. (1991). Physical activity and health enhancement in older adults: Current status and future prospects. *Annals of Behavioral Medicine, 13,* 87–90.

King, A. C., Haskell, W. L., Taylor, C. B., Kraemer, H. C., & DeBusk, R. F. (1991). Group- vs home-based exercise training in healthy older men and women. *Journal of the American Medical Association, 266,* 1535–1542.

King, A. C., Taylor, C. B., Haskell, W. L., & DeBusk, R. F. (1989). Influence of regular aerobic exercise on psychological health: A randomized, controlled trial of healthy middle-aged adults. *Health Psychology, 8,* 305–324.

King, A. C., Taylor, C. B., & Haskell, W. L. (1993). Effects of differing intensities and formats of 12 months of exercise training on psychological outcomes in older adults. *Health Psychology, 12,* 405.

King, M. B., Judge, J. O., Whipple, R. H., & Wolfson, L. (1993). Functional base of support improves with balance training. *Clinical Research, 41,* 220.

Kippenbrock, T., & Soja, M. E. (1993). Preventing falls in the elderly: Interviewing patients who have fallen. *Geriatric Nursing, 14,* 205–209.

Kirwan, J. P., Kohrt, W. M., Wojta, D. M., Bourey, R. E., & Holloszy, J. O. (1993). Endurance exercise training reduces glucose-stimulated insulin levels in 60- to 70-year-old men and women. *Journal of Gerontology: Medical Sciences, 48*(3), M84–M90.

Kohl, H. W., Gordon, N. F., Villegas, J. A., & Blair, S. N. (1992). Cardiorespiratory fitness, glycemic status, and mortality risk in men. *Diabetes Care, 15,* 184–192.

Kohrt, W. M., Malley, M. T., Coggan, A. R., Spina, R. J., Ogawa, T., Ehsani, A. A., Bourey, R. E., Martin, W. H., & Holloszy, J. O. (1991). Effects of gender, age, and fitness level on response of VO2max to training in 60 to 71 year olds. *Journal of Applied Physiology, 71,* 2004–2011.

Kohrt, W. M., Malley, M. T., Dalsky, G. P., & Holloszy, J. O. (1992). Body composition of healthy sedentary and trained young and older men and women. *Medicine & Science in Sports, 24,* 832–837.

Kohrt, W. M., Obert, K. A., & Holloszy, J. O. (1992). Exercise training improves fat distribution patterns in 60- to 70-year-old men and women. *Journal of Gerontology: Medical Sciences, 47*(4), M99–M105.

Koiso, T., & Ohsawa, S. (1992). Analysis of survival rates of sportsmen utilizing Cutler-Ederer method. *Journal of Human Ergology, 21*, 135–151.

Konradsen, L., Hansen, E. M., & Sondergaard, L. (1990). Long distance running and osteoarthrosis. *The American Journal of Sports Medicine, 18*, 379–381.

Kovar, P. A., Allegrante, J. P., MacKenzie, C. R., Peterson, M. G., Gutin, B., & Harlson, M. E. (1992). Supervised fitness walking in patients with osteoarthritis of the knee. A randomized, controlled trial. *Annals of Internal Medicine, 116*, 529–534.

Krall, E. A., & Dawson-Hughes, B. (1994). Walking is related to bone density and rates of bone loss. *American Journal of Medicine, 96*, 20–26.

Krause, N. (1993). Neighborhood deterioration and social isolation in later life. *International Journal of Aging & Human Development, 36*, 9–38.

Krause, N., Goldenhar, L., Liang, J., Jay, G. M., & Maeda, D. (1993). Stress and exercise among the Japanese elderly. *Social Science & Medicine, 36*, 1429–1441.

LaCroix, A. Z., Guralnik, J. M., Berkman, L. F., Wallace, R. B., & Satterfield, S. (1993). Maintaining mobility in later life. II. Smoking, alcohol consumption, physical activity, and body mass index. *American Journal of Epidemiology, 137*, 858–869.

Lahatta, E. (1993). Cardiovascular regulatory mechanisms in advanced age. *Physiological Reviews, 73*, 2.

Landers, D. M., & Petruzzello, S. J. (1994). Physical activity, fitness and anxiety. In C. Bouchard, R. Shephard, & T. Stephens (Eds.), *Physical activity, fitness and health*. Champaign, IL: Human Kinetics.

Lane, N. E., Bloch, D. A., Hubert, H. B., Jones, H., Simpson, U., & Fries, J. F. (1990). Running, osteoarthritis, and bone density: initial 2-year longitudinal study. *American Journal of Medicine, 88*, 452–459.

Lane, N. E., Bloch, D. A., Wood, P. D., & Fries, J. F. (1987). Aging, long-distance running and the development of musculoskeletal disability. *American Journal of Medicine, 82*, 772–780.

Lane, N. E., Michel, B., Bjorkengren, A., Oehlert, J., Shi, H., Bloch, D. A., & Fries, J. F. (1993). The risk of osteoarthritis with running and aging: a 5-year longitudinal study. *Journal of Rheumatology, 20*, 461–468.

Lau, E. M., Woo, J., Leung, P. C., Swaminathan, R., & Leung, D. (1992). The effects of calcium supplementation and exercise on bone density in elderly Chinese women. *Osteoporosis International, 2*, 168–173.

Leigh, J. P., & Fries, J. F. (1992). Health habits, health care use and costs in a sample of retirees. *Inquiry, 29*, 44–54.

Leigh, J. P., & Fries, J. F. (1993). Associations among healthy habits, age, gender, and education in a sample of retirees. *International Journal of Aging & Human Development, 36*, 139–155.

Leveille, S. G., LaCroix, A. Z., Hecht, J. A., Grothaus, L. C., & Wagner, E. H. (1993). Does walking decrease the risk for cardiovascular disease hospitalizations and all-cause mortality in older adults? Poster presented at the 46th Gerontological Society of America Annual Scientific Meetings, New Orleans, November.

Levi, F., LaVecchia, C., Negri, E., & Franceschi, S. (1993). Selected physical activities and the risk of endometrial cancer. *British Journal of Cancer, 67*, 846–851.

Lichenstein, M. L., Shields, S. L., Shiavi, R. G., & Burger, C. (1989). Exercise and balance in aged women: A pilot controlled clinical trial. *Archives of Physical Medicine & Rehabilitation, 70*, 138–143.

Lindsted, K. D., Tonstad, S., & Kuzma, J. W. (1991). Self-report of physical activity and patterns of mortality in seventh-day adventist men. *Journal of Clinical Epidemiology, 44*, 355–364.

Lobstein, D. D., Rasmussen, C. L., Dunphy, G. E., & Dunphy, M. J. (1989). Beta-endorphin and components of depression as powerful discriminators between joggers and sedentary middle-aged men. *Journal of Psychosomatic Research, 33*, 293–305.

Lokey, E. A., & Tran, Z. V. (1989). Effects of exercise training on serum lipid and lipoprotein concentrations in women: A meta-analysis. *International Journal of Sports Medicine, 10*(6), 424–429.

Loomis, R. A., & Thomas, C. D. (1991). Elderly women in nursing home and independent residence: Health, body attitudes, self-esteem and life satisfaction. *Canadian Journal on Aging, 10*, 224–231.

Lord, S. R., Caplan, G. A., Colagiuri, R., Colagiuri, S., & Ward, J. A. (1993). Sensorimotor function in older persons with diabetes. *Diabetic Medicine, 10*, 614–618.

Lord, S. R., Caplan, G. A., & Ward, J. A. (1993). Balance, reaction time, and muscle strength in exercising and nonexercising older women: A pilot study. *Archives of Physical Medicine & Rehabilitation, 74*, 837–839.

Lord, S. R., & Castell, S. (1994). Physical activity program for older persons: Effect on balance, strength, neuromuscular control, and reaction time. *Archives of Physical Medicine & Rehabilitation, 75*, 648–652.

Lord, S. R., Clark, R. D., & Webster, I. W. (1991a). Postural stability and associated physiological factors in a population of aged persons. *Journal of Gerontology: Medical Sciences, 46*(3), M69–76.

Lord, S. R., Clark, R. D., & Webster, I. W. (1991b). Physiological factors associated with falls in an elderly population. *Journal of the American Geriatric Society, 39*, 1194–1200.

Lord, S. R., Ward, J. A., Williams, P., & Anstey, K. J. (1993). An epidemiological study of falls in older community-dwelling women: The Randwick falls and fractures study. *Australian Journal of Public Health, 17*, 240–245.

Luotola, H. (1983). Blood pressure and hemodynamics in postmenopausal women during estradiol-17 beta substitution. *Annals of Clinical Research, 15 Suppl.*(38), 1–121.

Lupinacci, N. S., Rikli, R. E., Jones, C. J., & Ross, D. (1993). Age and physical activity effects on reaction time and digit symbol substitution performance in cognitively active adults. *Research Quarterly, 64*, 144–150.

Mace, N. (1987). Principles of activities for persons with dementia. *Physical & Occupational Therapy in Geriatrics, 5*, 13–27.

MacLennan, W. J., Hall, M. R., Timothy, J. I., & Robinson, M. (1980). Is weakness in old age due to muscle wasting? *Age & Ageing, 9*(3), 188–192.

MacNeil, R. D. (1988). Leisure programs and services for older adults: Past, present and future research. *Therapeutic Recreation Journal, 1*, 24–35.

MacRae, P. G., Feltner, M. E., & Reinsch, S. (1994). A 1-year exercise program for older women: Effects on falls, injuries, and physical performance. *Journal of Aging & Physical Activity, 2*, 127–142.

Madden, D. J., Blumenthal, J. A., & Allen, P. A. (1989). Improving aerobic capacity in healthy older adults does not necessarily lead to improved cognitive performance. *Psychology & Aging, 4*, 307–320.

Maki, B. E., Holliday, P. J., & Topper, A. K. (1991). Fear of falling and postural performance in the elderly. *Journal of Gerontology: Medical Sciences, 46*(4), M123–131.

Makrides, L., Heigenhauser, G. J., & Jones, N. L. (1986). High-intensity endurance training in 20–30 and 60- to 70 year-old men. *Journal of Applied Physiology, 69*(5), 1792–1798.

Malmivaara, A., Heliovaara, M., Knekt, P., Reunanen, A., & Aromaa, A. (1993). Risk factors for injurious falls leading to hospitalization or death in a cohort of 19,500 adults. *American Journal of Epidemiology, 138*, 384–394.

Marin, W. H., Ogawa, T., Kohrt, W. M., Malley, M. T., Korte, E., Kieffer, P. S., & Schechtman, K. B. (1991). Effects of aging, gender, and physical training on peripheral vascular function. *Circulation, 84*, 654–664.

Marti, B., Salonen, J., Tuomilhto, J., & Puska, P. (1988). 10-year trends in physical activity in the eastern Finnish population: Relationship to socioeconomic and lifestyle considerations. *Acta Medica Scandinavica, 224*, 195–203.

Martin, D., & Notelovitz, M. (1993). Effects of aerobic training on bone mineral density of postmenopausal women. *Journal of Bone & Mineral Research, 8*, 931–936.

Martin, III, W. H., Ogawa, T., Kohrt, W. M., Malley, M. T., Korte, E., Kieffer, P. S., & Schechtman, K. B. (1991). Effects of aging, gender, and physical training on peripheral vascular function. *Circulation, 84*, 654–664.

Mattar, J. A., Salas, C. E., Bernstein, D. P., Lehr, D., & Bauer, R. (1990). Hemodynamic changes after an intensive short-term exercise and nutrition program in hypertensive and obese patients with and without coronary artery disease. *Arquivos Brasileiros de Cardiologia, 54*, 307–312.

Mayer, J. A., Jermanovich, A., Wright, B. L., Elder, J. P., Drew, J. A., & Williams, S. J. (1994). Changes in health behaviors of older adults: The San Diego Medicare Preventive Health Project. *Preventive Medicine, 23*, 127–133.

Mayo, N. E., & Korner-Bitensky, N. (1993). Risk factors for fractures due to falls. *Archives of Physical Medicine & Rehabilitation, 74*, 917–921.

McAllister, R., & Broeder, C. E. (1993). Wellness strategies help workers adopt healthy habits in lifestyles. *Occupational Health & Safety, August*, 50, 52, 54, 56–58, 60.

McAuley, E. (1991). Efficacy, attributional, and affective responses to exercise participation. *Journal of Sport & Exercise Psychology, 13*, 382–393.

McAuley, E. (1992). The role of efficacy cognitions in the prediction of exercise behavior in middle-aged adults. *Journal of Behavioral Medicine, 15*, 65–88.

McAuley, E., & Courneya, K. S. (1992). Self-efficacy relationships with affective and exertion responses to exercise. *Journal of Applied Social Psychology, 22*, 312–326.

McAuley, E., Courneya, K. S., & Lettunich, J. (1991). Effects of acute and long-term exercise on self-efficacy responses in sedentary, middle-aged males and females. *The Gerontologist, 31*, 534–542.

McAuley, E., Lox, C., & Duncan, T. E. (1993). Long-term maintenance of exercise, self-efficacy, and physiological change in older adults. *Journal of Gerontology: Psychological Sciences, 48*, P218–P224.

McElvaney, G. N., Blackie, S. P., Morrison, N. J., Fairbarn, M. S., Wilcox, P. G., & Pardy, R. L. (1989). Cardiac output at rest and in exercise in elderly subjects. *Medicine and Science in Sports and Exercise, 21*, 293–298.

McMurdo, M. E., & Rennie, L. (1993). A controlled trial of exercise by residents of old people's homes. *Age & Ageing, 22,* 11–15.

McMurdo, M. E. T., & Burnett, L. (1992). Randomised controlled trial of exercise in the elderly. *Gerontology, 38,* 292–298.

McMurdo, M. E. T., & Rennie, L. M. (1994). Improvements in quadriceps strength with regular seated exercise in the institutionalized elderly. *Archives of Physical Medicine & Rehabilitation, 75,* 600–603.

McNeil, J. K., LeBlanc, E. M., & Joyner, M. (1991). The effect of exercise on depressive symptoms in the moderately depressed elderly. *Psychology & Aging, 6,* 487–488.

Meddaugh, D. I. (1987). Exercise-to-music for the abusive patient. In T. L. Brink (Ed.), *The elderly uncooperative patient* (pp. 147–153). New York: Haworth.

Meeuwsen, H. J., Sawicki, T. M., & Stelmach, G. E. (1993). Improved foot position sense as a result of repetitions in older adults. *Journal of Gerontology: Psychological Sciences, 48,* P137–141.

Mellemgaard, A., Engholm, G., McLaughlin, J. K., & Olsen, J. H. (1994). Risk factors for renal-cell carcinoma in Denmark, III. Role of weight, physical activity and reproductive factors. *International Journal of Cancer, 56,* 66–71.

Meyer, C. L., & Hawley, D. J. (1994). Characteristics of participants in water exercise programs compared to patients seen in a rheumatic disease clinic. *Arthritis Care & Research, 7,* 85–89.

Minor, M. A., & Brown, J. D. (1993). Exercise maintenance of persons with arthritis after participation in a class experience. *Health Education Quarterly, 20,* 83–95.

Minor, M. A., Hewett, J. E., Webel, R. R., Anderson, S. K., & Kay, D. R. (1989). Efficacy of physical conditioning exercise in patients with rheumatoid arthritis and osteoarthritis. *Arthritis & Rheumatism, 32(11),* 1396–1405.

Misner, J. E., Massey, B. H., Bemben, M., Going, S., & Patrick, J. (1992). Long-term effects of exercise on the range of motion of aging women. *Journal of Orthopaedic & Sports Physical Therapy, 16,* 37–42.

Mittleman, K., Crawford, S., Holliday, S., Gutman, G., & Bhaktan, G. (1989). The older cyclist: Anthropometric, physiological, and psychological changes observed during a trans-Canada cycle tour. *Canadian Journal on Aging, 8,* 144–156.

Mittleman, M. A., Maclure, M., Tofler, G. H., Sherwood, J. B., Goldberg, R. J., & Muller, J. E. (1993). Triggering of acute myocardial infarction by heavy physical exertion. Protection against triggering by regular exertion. *New England Journal of Medicine, 329,* 1677–1683.

Molloy, D. W., Beerschoten, D. A., Borrie, M. J., Crilly, R. G., & Cape, R. D. T. (1988). Acute effects of exercise on neuropsychological function in elderly subjects. *Journal of the American Geriatric Society, 36,* 29–33.

Molloy, D. W., Delaquerriere Richardson, L., & Crilly, R. G. (1988). The effects of a three-month exercise programme on neurophysiological function in elderly institutionalized women: A randomized controlled trial. *Age & Ageing, 17,* 303–310.

Morris, J. N., Clayton, D. G., Everitt, M. G., Semmence, A. M., & Burgess, E. H. (1990). Exercise in leisure time: Coronary attack and death rates. *British Heart Journal, 63,* 325–334.

Morris, R., Digenio, A., Padayachee, G. N., & Kinnear, B. (1993). The effect of a 6-month cardiac rehabilitation programme on serum lipoproteins and apoproteins A1 and B and lipoprotein a. *South African Medical Journal, 83,* 315–318.

Moskowitz, R. W., Howell, D. S., Goldberg, V. M., & Mankin, H. J. (1992). *Osteoarthritis: Diagnosis and medical surgical management*. Philadelphia: W. B. Saunders Company.

Mulrow, C. D., Gerety, M. B., Kanten, D., Cornell, J. E., DeNino, L. A., Chiodo, L., Aguilar, C., O'Neil, M. B., Rosenberg, J., & Solis, R. M. (1994). A randomized trial of physical rehabilitation for very frail nursing home residents. *Journal of the American Medical Association, 271*, 519–524.

Mummery, K. (1994). Is the message getting across? The definitial effectiveness of the Active Living slogan. *Research Update*, Alberta Centre for Well-Being, *1*(7), 1.

Myers, A. H., Baker, S. P., Van Natta, M. L., Abbey, H., & Robinson, E. G. (1991). Risk factors associated with falls and injuries among elderly institutionalized persons. *American Journal of Epidemiology, 133*, 1179–1190.

Myers, A. M., & Hamilton, N. (1985). Evaluation of the Canadian Red Cross Society's Fun and Fitness Program for seniors. *Canadian Journal on Aging, 4*, 201–212.

National Advisory Council on Aging (NACA). (1990). *Getting acquainted*. Brochure. Ottawa: Minister of Supply and Services.

National Advisory Council on Aging (1993). *The NACA position on women's life course events*. Ottawa: Minister of Supply and Services.

National Advisory Council on Aging. (1994). *Healthy choices for healthy aging*. Otttawa: Minister of Supply and Services.

Nelson, M. E., Fisher, E. C., Dilmanian, F. A., Dallal, G. E., & Evans, W. J. (1991). A 1-year walking program and increased dietary calcium in postmenopausal women: Effects on bone. *The American Journal of Clinical Nutrition, 53*, 1304–1311.

Nevitt, M. C., Cummings, S. R., & Hudes, E. S. (1991). Risk factors for injurious falls: A prospective study. *Journal of Gerontology: Medical Sciences, 46*(5), M164–M170.

Nieman, D. C., Henson, D. A., Gusewitch, G., Warren, B. J., Dotson, R. C., Butterworth, D. E., & Nehlsen-Cannarella, S. L. (1993). Physical activity and immune function in elderly women. *Medicine & Science in Sports, 25*, 823–831.

Nieman, D. C., Pover, N. K., Segebartt, K. S., Arabatzis, K., Johnson, M., & Dietrich, S. J. (1990). Hematological, anthropometric, and metabolic comparisons between active and inactive healthy elderly women. *Annals of Sports Medicine, 5*, 2–8.

Nieman, D. C., Warren, B. J., O'Donnell, K. A., Dotson, R. G., Butterworth, D. E., & Henson, D. A. (1993). Physical activity and serum lipids and lipoproteins in elderly women. *Journal of the American Geriatric Society, 41*, 1339–1344.

Normand, R., Kerr, R., & Metivier, G. (1987). Exercise, aging and fine motor performance: An assessment. *The Journal of Sports Medicine & Physical Fitness, 27*, 488–496.

Norvell, N., Martin, D., & Salamon, A. (1991). Psychological and physiological benefits of passive and aerobic exercise in sedentary middle-aged women. *Journal of Mental and Nervous Disease, 179*, 573–574.

Novak, M. (1994). Access to active living for seniors. *Access to active living proceedings* (pp. 1–11). 10th Commonwealth and International Scientific Conference, University of Victoria, Victoria, B.C., August, 10–14, 1994.

O'Brien Cousins, S. (1993). The determinants of late life exercise in women over age 70. Unpublished doctoral dissertation. Department of Administrative, Adult and Higher Education. The University of British Columbia, Vancouver, B.C.

O'Brien Cousins, S. (1995). Social support for exercise among elderly women in Canada. *Health Promotion International, 10*(4), 273–282.

O'Brien Cousins, S. (1996) . Exercise cognition among elderly women. *Journal of Applied Sport Psychology, 8*(2), 131–145.

O'Brien Cousins, S. (1997). Elderly tomboys? Self-efficacy for physical activity may originate in childhood. *Journal of Aging & Physical Activity, 5*, 229–243.

O'Brien Cousins, S., & Burgess, A. C. (1992). Perspectives on older adults in sport and physical activity. *Educational Gerontology, 18*, 461–481.

O'Brien Cousins, S. J., & Keating, N. (1995). Life cycle patterns of physical activity among sedentary and active older women. *Journal of Aging & Physical Activity, 3*, 340–359.

O'Brien Cousins, S. J., & Vertinsky, P. A. (1995). Recapturing the physical activity experiences of the old: A study of three women. *Journal of Aging & Physical Activity, 3*, 146–162.

O'Donnell, D. E., Webb, K. A., & McGuire, M. A. (1993). Older patients with COPD: Benefits of exercise training. *Geriatrics, 48*, 60–66.

Ogawa, T., Spina, R. J., Martin, W. H., Kohrt, W. M., Schechtman, K. B., Holloszy, T. O., & Ehsani, A. A. (1992). Effects of aging, sex and physical training on cardiovascular response to exercise. *Circulation, 86*, 494–503.

O'Hagan, C. M., Smith, D. M., & Pileggi, K. L. (1994). Exercise classes in rest homes: Effect on physical function. *New Zealand Medical Journal, 107*, 39–40.

Oldridge, N. B., & Rogowski, B. L. (1990). Self-efficacy and in-patient cardiac rehabilitation. *The American Journal of Cardiology, 66*, 362–365.

O'Loughlin, J. L., Robitaille, Y., Boivin, J. F., & Suissa, S. (1993). Incidence of and risk factors for falls and injurious falls among the community dwelling elderly. *American Journal of Epidemiology, 137*, 342–354.

Orban, W. A. R. (1994). Active living for older adults: A model for optimal living. In H. A. Quinney, L. Gauvin, & A. E. Wall (Eds.), *Toward active living* (pp. 153–161). Champaign, IL: Human Kinetics.

Ory, M. G., Schechtman, K. B., Miller, J. P., Hadley, E. C., Fiatarone, M. A., Province, M. A., Arfken, C. L., Morgan, D., Weiss, S., & Kaplan, M. (1993). Frailty and injuries in later life: The FICSIT trials. *Journal of the American Geriatric Society, 41*, 283–296.

Ostrow, A. C., & Dzewaltowski, D. A. (1986). Older adults' perceptions of physical activity participation based on age-role and sex-role appropriateness. *Research Quarterly for Exercise & Sport, 57*(20), 167–169.

Paez, P. N., Phillipson, E. A., Masangkay, M., & Sproule, B. J. (1967). The physiologic basis of training patients with emphysema. *American Review of Respiratory Disease, 95*, 944.

Paffenbarger, R. S. J., Hyde, R. T., & Wing, A. L. (1993). Changes in physical-activity level and long-term mortality in men. *Clinical Journal of Sports Medicine, 3*.

Paffenbarger, R. S., Jr., Hyde, R. T., Wing, A. L., Lee, I. M., Jung, J. L., & Kampert, J. B. (1993). The association of changes in physical activity level and other lifestyle characteristics with mortality among men. *New England Journal of Medicine, 328*, 538–545.

Page, R. C. L., Harnden, K. E., Walravens, N. K. N., Onslow, C., Sutton, P., Levy, J. C., Hockaday, D. T. R., & Turner, R. C. (1993). 'Healthy living' and sulphonylurea therapy have different effects on glucose tolerance and risk factors for vascular disease in subjects with impaired glucose tolerance. *Quarterly Journal of Medicine, 86*, 145–154.

Palmer, J., Vace, N., & Epstein, J. (1988). Adult inpatient alcoholics: Physical exercise as a treatment intervention. *Journal of Studies on Alcohol, 49*, 418–421.

Panton, L. B., Graves, J. E., Pollock, M. L., Hagberg, J. M., & Chen, W. (1990). Effect of aerobic and resistance training on fractionated reaction time and speed of movement. *Journal of Gerontology: Medical Sciences, 45*(1), M26–M31.

Perri, II, S., & Templar, D. I. (1984–1985). The effects of an aerobic exercise program on psychological variables in older adults. *International Journal of Aging & Human Development, 20,* 167–172.

Petersen, M. G. E., Kovar-Toledano, P. A., Allegrante, J. P., Mackenzie, E. R., Gutin, B., & Kroll, M. A. (1993). Effect of a walking program on gait characteristics in patients with arthritis. *Arthritis Care & Research, 6,* 11–15.

Petrella, R. J., Cunningham, D. A., & Smith, J. J. (1989). Influence of age and physical training on postural adaptation. *Canadian Journal of Sport Science, 14,* 4–9.

Petruzzello, S. J., Landers, D. M., Hatfield, B. D., Kubitz, K. A., & Salazar, W. (1991). A meta-analysis on the anxiety-reducing effects of acute and chronic exercise. Outcomes and mechanisms. *Sports Medicine, 11,* 143–182.

Pollock, M. L., Carroll, J. F., Graves, J. E., Leggett, S. H., Braith, R. W., Limacher, M., & Hagberg, J. M. (1991). Injuries and adherence to walk/jog and resistance training programs in the elderly. *Medicine & Science in Sports, 23,* 1194–2000.

Posner, J. D., Gorman, K. M., Windsor-Lansberg, L., Larsen, J., Bleiman, M., Shaw, C., Rosenberg, B., & Knebl, J. (1992). Low to moderate intensity endurance training in healthy older adults: Physiological responses after four months. *Journal of the American Geriatric Society, 40,* 1–7.

Powell, R. R. (1974). Psychological effects of exercise therapy upon geriatric mental patients. *Journal of Gerontology, 29,* 157–161.

Powell, K., Thompson, P., Caspersen, C., & Kendrick, J. (1987). Physical activity and the incidence of coronary heart disease. *Public Health Reports, 101,* 15–21.

Puggaard, L., Pedersen, H. P., Sandager, E., & Klitgaard, H. (1994). Physical conditioning in elderly people. *Scandinavian Journal of Medicine, Science, & Sports, 4,* 47–56.

Pukkala, E., Poskiparta, M., Apter, D., & Vihko, V. (1993). Life-long physical activity and cancer risk among Finnish female teachers. *European Journal of Cancer Prevention, 2,* 369–376.

Pyka, G., Lindenberger, E., Charette, S., & Marcus, R. (1994). Muscle strength and fiber adaptations to a year-long resistance training program in elderly men and women. *Journal of Gerontology, 49*(1), M22–M27.

Quinn, T. J., Sprague, H. A., Van Huss, W. D., & Olson, H. W. (1990). Caloric expenditure, life status, and disease in former male athletes and non-athletes. *Medicine & Science in Sports, 22,* 742–750.

Ragheb, M. G., & Griffith, C. A. (1982). The contribution of leisure participation and leisure satisfaction to life satisfaction of older persons. *Journal of Leisure Research, 14,* 295–306.

Ragosta, M., Crabtree, J., Sturner, W. Q., & Thompson, P. D. (1984). Death during recreational exercise in the state of Rhode Island. *Medicine & Science in Sports & Exercise, 16*(4), 339–342.

Rakowski, W., & Mor, V. (1992). The association of physical activity with mortality among older adults in the Longitudinal Study of Aging. *Journal of Gerontology: Medical Sciences, 47*(4), M122–M129.

Rantanen, T., Era, P., Kauppinen, M., & Heikkinen, E. (1994). Maximal isometric muscle strength and socio-economic status, health, and physical activity in 75-year-old persons. *Journal of Aging & Physical Activity, 2,* 206–220.

Rantanen, T., Parkatti, T., & Heikkinen, E. (1992). Muscle strength according to level of physical exercise and educational background in middle-aged women in Finland. *European Journal of Applied Physiology, 65*, 507–512.

Reaven, P. D., Barrett-Connor, E., & Edelstein, S. (1991). Relation between leisure-time physical activity and blood pressure in older women. *Circulation, 83*, 559–565.

Rehm, J., Fichter, M. M., & Elton, M. (1993). Effects on mortality of alcohol consumption, smoking, physical activity, and close personal relationships. *Addiction, 88*, 101–112.

Reinsch, S., MacRae, P., Lachenbruch, P. A., & Tobis, J. S. (1992). Attempts to prevent falls and injury: A prospective community study. *The Gerontologist, 32*, 450–456.

Reuben, D. B., Laliberte, L., Hiris, J., & Mor, V. (1990). A hierarchical exercise scale to measure function at the Advanced Activities of Daily Living (AADL) level. *Journal of the American Geriatric Society, 38*, 855–861.

Riddick, C. C., & Daniel, S. N. (1984). The relative contribution of leisure activities and other factors to the mental health of older women. *Journal of Leisure Research, 16*, 136–148.

Rider, R. A., & Daly, J. (1991). Effects of flexibility training on enhancing spinal mobility in older women. *The Journal of Sports Medicine & Physical Fitness, 31*, 213–217.

Rikli, R. E., & Edwards, D. J. (1991). Effects of a three-year exercise program on motor function and cognitive processing speed in older women. *Research Quarterly, 62*, 61–67.

Rikli, R. E., & McManis, B. G. (1990). Effects of exercise on bone mineral content in postmenopausal women. *Research Quarterly, 61*, 243–249.

Roberts, B. L. (1989). Effects of walking on balance among elders. *Nursing Research, 38*, 180–182.

Roberts, B. L. (1990). Effects of walking on reaction and movement times among elders. *Perceptual & Motor Skills, 71*, 131–140.

Robinson, S. (1938). Experimental studies of physical fitness in relation to age. *Arbeitphysiologie, 10*, 223–251.

Rodeheffer, R. J., Gerstenblith, G., Becher, L. C., Fleg, J. L., Weisfeldt, M., & Lahatta, E. G. (1984). Exercise cardiac output is maintained with advancing age in healthy human subjects: Cardiac dilitation and increased stroke volume compensate for a diminished heart rate. *Circulation, 69*(2), 203–213.

Rogers, M. A. (1989). Acute effects of exercise on glucose tolerance in non-insulin dependent diabetics. *Medicine and Science in Sports and Exercise*, 362–368.

Rogers, M. A., Hagberg, J. M., Martin, III, W. H., Ehsani, A. A., & Holloszy, J. O. (1990). Decline in VO_2max with aging in master athletes and sedentary men. *Journal of Applied Physiology, 68*, 2195–2199.

Rogers, R. L., Meyer, J. S., & Mortel, K. F. (1990). After reaching retirement age physical activity sustains cerebral perfusion and cognition. *Journal of the American Geriatric Society, 38*, 123–128.

Rooney, E. M. (1993). Exercise for older patients: Why it's worth your effort. *Geriatrics, 48*, 68, 71–74, 77.

Roth, D. L. (1989). Acute emotional and psychological effects of aerobic exercise. *Psychophysiology, 26*, 694–701.

Rotter, J. B. (1966). Generalized expectancies for internal versus external control of reinforcement. *Journal of Consulting & Clinical Psychology, 43*, 56–67.

Ruderman, N., Horton, E. S., & Kemmer, F. W. (1992). Introduction: Diabetes and exercise 1990. *Diabetes Care, 15*, 1676–1677.

Ruderman, N. B., & Schneider, S. H. (1992). Diabetes, exercise, and atherosclerosis. *Diabetes Care, 15,* 1787–1791.

Rudman, W. (1987). The social and psychological benefits of involvement in corporate programs through retirement. Special Issue: Family and economic issues. Diversity in the lifestyles of older people. *Lifestyles, 8,* 95–105, 225–235.

Rutherford, O. M., & Jones, D. A. (1992). The relationship of muscle and bone loss and activity levels with age in women. *Age & Ageing, 21,* 286–293.

Salonen, J., Slater, J., Tuomilhto, J., & Rauramaa, R. (1988). Leisure time and occupational physical activity: Risk of death from ischemic heart disease. *American Journal of Epidemiology, 127,* 87–94.

Salthouse, T. A. (1988). The role of processing resources in cognitive aging. In M. L. Lowe & C. J. Brainerd (Eds.), *Cognitive development in adulthood: Progress in cognitive development research* (pp. 185–240). New York: Springer.

Sandvik, L., Erikssen, J., Thaulow, E., Erikksen, G., Mundal, R., & Rodahl, K. (1993). Physical fitness as a predictor of mortality among healthy, middle-aged Norwegian men. *New England Journal of Medicine, 328,* 533–537.

Sarna, S., Sahi, T., Koskenvuo, M., & Kaprio, J. (1993). Increased life expectancy of world class male athletes. *Medicine & Science in Sports, 25,* 237–244.

Satariano, W. A., Ragheb, N. E., Branch, L. G., & Swanson, G. M. (1990). Difficulties in physical functioning reported by middle-aged and elderly women with breast cancer: a case-control comparison. *Journal of Gerontology, 45,* M3–11.

Sattin, R. W. (1992). Falls among older persons: A public health perspective. [review]. *Annual Review of Public Health, 13,* 489–508.

Sauvage, L. R. J., Myklebust, B. M., Crow-Pan, J., Novak, S., Millington, P., Hoffman, M. D., Hartz, A. J., & Rudman, D. (1992). A clinical trial of strengthening and aerobic exercise to improve gait and balance in elderly male nursing home residents. *American Journal of Physical Medicine & Rehabilitation, 71,* 333–342.

Schneider, S. H., Amorosa, L. F., Clemow, L., Khachadurian, A. V., & Ruderman, N. B. (1992). Ten-year experience with an exercise-based outpatient life-style modification program in the treatment of diabetes mellitus. *Diabetes Care, 15,* 1800–1809.

Schoenborn, C. A. (1993). The Alameda Study - 25 years later. *International Review of Health Psychology, 2,* 81–116.

Schroll, M. (1994). The main pathway to musculoskeletal disability. *Scandinavian Journal of Medicine, Science, & Sports, 4,* 3–12.

Seals, D. R., Hagberg, J. M., Hurley, B. F., Ehsani, A. A., & Holloszy, J. O. (1984). Endurance training in older men and women. I. Cardiovascular responses to exercise. *Journal of Applied Physiology, 57,* 1024–1029.

Seals, D. R., Hagberg, J. M., Hurley, B. F., Ehsani, A. A., & Holloszy, J. O. (1984). Effects of endurance training on glucose tolerance and plasma lipid levels in older men and women. *Journal of the American Medical Association, 252,* 645–649.

Sedgwick, A. W., Taplin, R. E., Davidson, A. H., & Thomas, D. W. (1988). Effects of physical activity on risk factors for coronary heart disease in previously sedentary women: A five-year longitudinal study. *Australia & New Zealand Journal of Medicine, 18,* 600–605.

Segebartt, K. S., Nieman, D. C., Pover, N. K., Arabatzis, K., & Johnson, M. (1988). Psychological well-being in physically active and inactive healthy young old to very old women. *Annals of Sports Medicine, 4,* 130–136.

Sharpe, P. A., & Connell, C. M. (1992). Exercise beliefs and behaviours among older employees: A health promotion trial. *The Gerontologist, 32,* 444–449.

Shay, K. A., & Roth, D. L. (1992). Association between aerobic fitness and visuospatial performance in healthy older adults. *Psychology & Aging, 7,* 15–24.

Shephard, R. J. (1989). Critical issues in the health of the elderly: The role of physical activity. *Canadian Journal on Aging, 3,* 199–207.

Shephard, R. J. (1992). Does exercise reduce all-cancer death rates? *British Journal of Sports Medicine, 26,* 125–128.

Shephard, R. J. (1993). Exercise and aging: Extending independence in older adults. *Geriatrics, 48,* 61–64.

Shephard, R. J. (1994). Physical activity and reduction of health risks: How far are the benefits independent of fat loss? *The Journal of Sports Medicine & Physical Fitness, 34,* 91–98.

Shephard, R. J., Berridge, M., Montelpare, W., Daniel, J. V., & Flowers, J. F. (1987). Exercise compliance of elderly volunteers. *The Journal of Sports Medicine & Physical Fitness, 27,* 410–418.

Shephard, R. J., Montelpare, W., Berridge, M., & Flowers, J. (1986). Influence of exercise and of lifestyle education upon attitudes to exercise of older people. *The Journal of Sports Medicine & Physical Fitness, 26,* 175–179.

Shu, X. O., Hatch, M. C., Zheng, W., Gao, Y. T., & Brinton, L. A. (1993). Physical activity and risk of endometrial cancer. *Epidemiology, 4,* 342–349.

Sidney, K. H., & Shephard, R. J. (1976). Attitudes towards health and physical activity in the elderly. Effects of a physical training program. *Medicine & Science in Sports, 8,* 246–252.

Simonsick, E. M., Lafferty, M. E., Phillips, C. L., Mendes de Leon, C. F., Kasl, S. V., Seeman, T. E., Fillenbaum, G., Hebert, P., & Lemke, J. H. (1993). Risk due to inactivity in physically capable older adults. *American Journal of Public Health, 83,* 1443–1450.

Singh, R. B., Singh, N. K., Rastogi, S. S., Mani, U. V., & Niaz, M. A. (1993). Effects of diet and lifestyle changes on atherosclerotic risk factors after 24 weeks on the Indian Diet Heart Study. *The American Journal of Cardiology, 71,* 1283–1288.

Siscovick, D. S. (1990). Exercise and sudden cardiac death: Is the run worth the risk? *Transactions of the Association of Life Insurance Medical Directors of America, 73,* 37–44.

Skarfors, E. T., Lithell, H., Silenius, I., & Wegener, T. A. (1987). Physical training as treatment for type II (non-insulin-dependent) diabetes in elderly men. *Diabetologia, 30,* 930–933.

Slattery, M. L., Abd-Elghany, N., Kerber, R., & Schumacher, M. C. (1990). Physical activity and colon cancer: A comparison of various indicators of physical activity to evaluate the association. *Epidemiology, 1,* 481–485.

Speake, D. L., Cowart, M. E., & Pellet, K. (1989). Health perceptions and lifestyles of the elderly. *Research in Nursing & Health, 12,* 93–100.

Speake, D. L., Cowart, M. E., & Stephens, R. (1991). Healthy lifestyle practices of rural and urban elderly. *Health Values, 15,* 45–51.

Speechly, M., & Tinetti, M. (1991). Falls and injuries in frail and vigorous community elderly persons. *Journal of the American Geriatric Society, 39,* 46–52.

Spina, R. J., Ogawa, T., Kohrt, W. M., Martin III, W. H., Holloszy, J. O., & Ehsani, A. A. (1993). Differences in cardiovascular adaptations to endurance exercise training between older men and women. *Journal of Applied Physiology, 75*, 849–855.

Spina, R. J., Ogawa, T., Miller, T. R., Kohrt, W. M., & Ehsani, A. A. (1993). Effect of exercise training on left ventricular performance in older women free of cardiopulmonary disease. *The American Journal of Cardiology, 71*, 99–104.

Stacey, C., Kozma, A., & Stones, M. J. (1985). Simple cognitive and behavioural changes resulting from improved physical fitness in persons over 50 years of age. *Canadian Journal on Aging, 4*, 67–74.

Stamford, B. A., Hambacher, W., & Fallica, A. (1974). Effects of daily physical exercise on the psychiatric state of institutionalized geriatric mental patients. *Research Quarterly, 45*, 34–41.

Steinhardt, M. A., & Young, D. R. (1992). Psychological attributes of participants and nonparticipants in a worksite health and fitness center. *Behavioral Medicine, 18*, 40–46.

Steinhaus, L. A., Dustman, R. E., Ruhling, R. O., Emmerson, R. Y., Johnson, S. C., Shearer, D. E., Latin, R. W., Shigeoka, J. W., & Bonekat, W. H. (1990). Aerobic capacity of older adults: A training study. *The Journal of Sports Medicine & Physical Fitness, 30*, 163–172.

Stelmach, G. E. (1994). Physical activity and aging: Sensory and perceptual processing. In C. Bouchard, R. J. Shepard, & T. Stephens (Eds.), *Physical activity, fitness and health: International proceedings and consensus statement* (pp. 509–510). Champaign, IL: Human Kinetics.

Stenstrom, C. H. (1994). Radiologically observed progression of joint destruction and its relationship with demographic factors, disease severity, and exercise frequency in patients with rheumatoid arthritis. *Physical Therapy, 74*, 32–39.

Stephens, T. (1987). Secular trends in adult physical activity: Exercise boom or bust? *Research Quarterly, 58*, 94–105.

Stephens, T. (1988). Physical activity and mental health in the United States and Canada: Evidence from four population surveys. *Preventive Medicine, 17*, 35–47.

Stephens, T., Craig, C. L., & Ferris, B. F. (1986). Adult physical activity in Canada: Findings from the Canadian Fitness Survey I. *Canadian Journal of Public Health, 77*, 285–290.

Stevenson, J., Tacia, S., Thompson, J., & Crane, C. (1988, May 28 Saturday). A comparison of land and water exercise programs for older individuals. *Medicine & Science in Sports & Exercise,* S90.

Stevenson, J. S., & Topp, R. (1990). Effects of moderate and low intensity long-term exercise by older adults. *Research in Nursing & Health, 13*, 209–218.

Stones, M. J., & Kozma, A. (1988). Physical activity, age, and cognitive/motor performance. In M. L. Howe & C. J. Brainerd (Eds.), *Cognitive development in adulthood, progress in cognitive development research* (pp. 273–321). New York, NY: Springer-Verlag.

Stones, M. J., & Kozma, A. (1989). Age, exercise, and coding performance. *Psychology & Aging, 4*, 190–194.

Studenski, S., Duncan, P. W., & Chandler, J. (1991). Postural responses and effector factors in persons with unexplained falls: Results and methodologic issues. *Journal of the American Geriatric Society, 39*, 229–234.

Sturgeon, S. R., Brinton, L. A., Berman, M. L., Mortel, R., Twiggs, L. B., Barrett, R. J., & Wilbanks, G. D. (1993). Past and present physical activity and endometrial cancer risk. *British Journal of Cancer, 68*, 584–589.

Sulman, J., & Wilkinson, S. (1989). An activity group for long-stay elderly patients in an acute care hospital: Program evaluation. *Canadian Journal on Aging, 8*, 34–50.

Suominen, H. (1993). Bone mineral density and long-term exercise: An overview of cross-sectional athlete studies. *Sports Medicine, 16*, 316–330.

Suominen, H., Heikkinen, E., & Parkatti, T. (1977). Effect of eight weeks' physical training on muscle and connective tissue of the m. vastus lateralis in 69-year-old men and women. *Journal of Gerontology, 32*, 33–37.

Suominen, H., & Rahkila, P. (1991). Bone mineral density of the calcaneus in 70- to 81-year-old male athletes and a population sample. *Medicine & Science in Sports, 23*, 1227–1233.

Svanstrom, L. (1990). Simply osteoporosis - or multifactorial genesis for the increasing incidence of fall injuries in the elderly? *Scandinavian Journal of Social Medicine, 18*, 165–169.

Swerts, P. M. J., Kretzers, L. M. J., Terpstra-Lindeman, E., Verstappen, F. T. J., & Wouters, E. F. M. (1990). Exercise reconditioning in the rehabilitation of patients with chronic obstructive pulmonary disease: A short- and long-term analysis. *Archives of Physical Medicine & Rehabilitation, 71*, 570–573.

Takeshima, N., Tanaka, K., Kobayashi, F., Watanabe, T., & Kato, T. (1993). Effects of aerobic exercise conditioning at intensities corresponding to lactate threshold in the elderly. *European Journal of Applied Physiology, 67*, 138–143.

Taylor, A. W. (1992). Aging: A normal degenerative process — with or without regular exercise. *Canadian Journal of Sport Science, 17*, 163–167.

Taylor, J. (1995). How to overload the health care system. *Active Living, 4*(3), 1–2.

Taylor, J. (1996). Why time is running out for Canada's baby boomers. *Active Living, 5*(2), 1–2, 5.

Teasdale, N., Stelmach, G. E., & Breunig, A. (1991). Postural sway characteristics of the elderly under normal and altered visual and support surface conditions. *Journal of Gerontology: Biological Sciences, 46*, B238–B244.

Teno, J., Kiel, D. P., & Mor, V. (1990). Multiple stumbles: A risk factor for falls in community-dwelling elderly: A prospective study. *Journal of the American Geriatric Society, 38*, 1321–1325.

Thomas, S. G., Weller, I., & Cox, M. H. (1993). Sources of variation in oxygen consumption during a stepping task. *Medicine and Science in Sports and Exercise, 25*, 139–144.

Ting, A. J. (1991). Running and the older athlete. *Clinics in Geriatric Medicine, 10*, 319–325.

Topp, R., Mikesky, A., Wigglesworth, J., Holt, W., & Edwards, J. E. (1993). The effect of a 12-week dynamic resistance strength training program on gait velocity and balance of older adults. *The Gerontologist, 33*, 501–506.

Topper, A. K., Maki, B. E., & Holliday, P. J. (1993). Are activity-based assessments of balance and gait in the elderly predictive of risk of falling and/or type of fall? *Journal of the American Geriatric Society, 41*, 479–487.

Toshima, M. T., Kaplan, R. M., & Ries, A. L. (1990). Experimental evaluation of rehabilitation in chronic obstructive pulmonary disease: Short-term effects on exercise endurance and health status. *Health Psychology, 9*, 237–252.

Tucker, L. A., & Mortell, R. (1993). Comparison of the effects of walking and weight training programs on body image in middle-aged women: An experimental study. *American Journal of Health Promotion, 8*, 34–42.

U.S. Department of Health and Human Services (USDHHS). (1994). *Health United States 1993*. Public Health Service: Hyattsville, MD.

Valliant, P. M., & Asu, M. E. (1985). Exercise and its effects on cognition and physiology in older adults. *Perceptual & Motor Skills, 61*, 1031–1038.

Van Camp, S. P. (1988). Exercise-related sudden death: risks and causes. *The Physician & Sportsmedicine, 16*(5), 97–109.

Van Camp, S. P., & Peterson, R. A. (1986). Cardiovascular complications of outpatient cardiac rehabilitation programs. *Journal of the American Medical Association, 256*, 1160–1163.

Vetter, R., Dosemeci, M., Blair, A., Wacholder, S., Unsal, M., Engin, K., & Fraumeni, J. F. J. (1992). Occupational physical activity and colon cancer risk in Turkey. *European Journal of Epidemiology, 8*, 845–850.

Volden, C., Langemo, D., Adamson, M., & Oechsle, L. (1990). The relationship of age, gender, and exercise practices to measures of health, life-style, and self-esteem. *Applied Nursing Research, 3*, 20–26.

Voorips, L. E., Lemmink, K. A., Van Heuvelen, M. J. G., Bult, P., & Van Staveren, W. A. (1993). The physical condition of elderly women differing in habitual physical activity. *Medicine & Science in Sports, 25*, 1152–1157.

Wagner, L. (1992). Non-institutional care for the elderly. A Danish model. *Danish Medical Bulletin, 39*, 236–238.

Wallberg-Henriksson, H. (1989). Acute exercise: Fuel homeostasis and glucose transport in insulin-dependent diabetes mellitus. *Medicine and Science in Sports and Exercise*, 356–360.

Wallston, K. A., & Wallston, B. S. (1978). Health locus of control. *Health Education Monographs, 6*(1), 100–105.

Wankel, L. M., Hills, C. A., Hudec, J. C., Mummery, W. K., Sefton, J. M., Stevenson, J., & Whitmarsh, B. (1994). Self-esteem and body image: Structure, formation and relationship to health-related behaviors. Unpublished report submitted to the Canadian Fitness of Lifestyle Research Institute. Department of Physical Education and Sport Studies. The University of Alberta, Edmonton, AB, Canada.

Wankel, L. M., & Sefton, J. M. (1993). Physical activity and other lifestyle behaviors. In *Physical activity, fitness and health: International proceedings and consensus statement* (pp. 530–550). Champaign, IL: Human Kinetics.

Warren, B. J., Nieman, D. C., Dotson, R. G., Adkins, C. H., O'Donnell, K. A., Haddock, B. L., & Butterworth, D. E. (1993). Cardiorespiratory responses to exercise training in septuagenarian women. *International Journal of Sports Medicine, 14*, 60–65.

Weaver, T. E., & Narsavage, G. L. (1992). Physiological and psychological variables related to functional status in chronic obstructive pulmonary disease. *Nursing Research, 41*, 286–291.

Webb, G. D., Poehlman, E. T., & Tonino, R. P. (1993). Dissociation of changes in metabolic rate and blood pressure with erythrocyte Na-K pump activity in older men after endurance training. *Journal of Gerontology: Medical Sciences, 48*(2), M47–M52.

Weber, F., Barnard, R. J., & Roy, D. (1983). Effects of a high-complex-carbohydrate, low-fat diet and daily exercise on individuals 70 years of age and older. *Journal of Gerontology, 38*, 155–161.

Weiner, D. K., Bongiorni, D. R., Studenski, S. A., Duncan, P. W., & Kochersberger, G. G. (1993). Does functional reach improve with rehabilitation? *Archives of Physical Medicine & Rehabilitation, 74*, 796–800.

Weinstein, L. B. (1986). The benefits of aquatic activity. *Journal of Gerontological Nursing, 12*, 7–11.

Whitehurst, M. (1991). Reaction time unchanged in older women following aerobic training. *Perceptual & Motor Skills, 72*, 251–256.

Whitehurst, M., & Menendez, E. (1991). Endurance training in older women: Lipid and lipoprotein responses. *The Physician & Sportsmedicine, 19*, 95–104.

Whitemore, A. S., Wu-Williams, A. H., Lee, M., Zheng, S., Gallagher, R. P., Jiao, D. A., Zhou, L., Wang, X. H., Chen, K., & Jung, D. (1990). Diet, physical activity, and colorectal cancer among Chinese in North America and China. *Journal of the National Cancer Institute, 82*, 915–926.

Whitley, J. D., & Schoene, L. L. (1987). Comparison of heart rate responses: Water walking versus treadmill walking. *Physical Therapy, 67*, 1501–1504.

Whittington, R. M., & Banerjee, A. (1994). Sport-related sudden natural death in the City of Birmingham. *Journal of the Royal Society of Medicine, 87*, 18–21.

Williams, M. (1987). Type 2 diabetes: A new emphasis for prevention and management? *ACHPER National Journal*, 13–15.

Wolfson, L., Whipple, R., Amerman, P., & Tobin, J. N. (1990). Gait assessment in the elderly: A gait abnormality rating scale and its relation to falls. *Journal of Gerontology: Medical Sciences, 45*(1), M12–M19.

Wolfson, L., Whipple, R., Derby, C. A., Amerman, P., & Nashner, L. (1994). Gender differences in the balance of healthy elderly as demonstrated by dynamic posturography. *Journal of Gerontology: Medical Sciences, 49*(4), M160–M167.

Wong, D. E., Rechnitzer, P. A., Cunningham, D. A., & Howard, J. H. (1990). Effect of an exercise program on the perception of exertion in males at retirement. *Canadian Journal of Sport Science, 15*, 249–253.

Index

sense of
and anxiety, 137
and cancer, 113
and strength training, 23
Coping. *See* Stress
Coronary heart disease (CHD)
and lipid/lipoprotein profiles, 35–36, 98–99
research outcomes on, 96–99, 100*t*–102*t*
sudden death from, 133–134
Correlational research, 12
activities of daily living, 185*t*–187*t*
anxiety outcomes, 145*t*
arthritis outcomes, 111*t*–112*t*
body composition outcomes, 43*t*–45*t*
bone health/osteoporosis, 106*t*–107*t*
cancer outcomes, 116*t*–118*t*
cognitive/psychomotor outcomes, 62*t*–63*t*
coronary heart disease outcomes, 102*t*
depression outcomes, 152*t*–153*t*
falls outcomes, 87*t*–89*t*
habitual physical activity outcomes, 177*t*
joint mobility outcomes, 33*t*
life satisfaction outcomes, 166*t*
lipid/lipoprotein profile outcomes, 43*t*–45*t*
locus of control outcomes, 164*t*
mortality outcomes, 125*t*–130*t*
muscular strength outcomes, 27*t*
nutrition outcomes, 43*t*–45*t*
obesity outcomes, 43*t*–45*t*
self-esteem outcomes, 157*t*
Cost-benefit research, on active living, 12, 191

Database production, for present review, 5–7
Deconditioning
and bone strength, loss of, 99–100
and muscular strength reduction, 22
Degenerative joint disease, obesity and, 38
Dementia, 3, 10
research outcomes on, 10, 95–96, 97*t*
Depression
and anxiety, of chronic obstructive pulmonary patients, 138
and coronary events, 184
and locus of control, 161
and mortality, 132
research outcomes on, 144–151, 146*t*–150*t*, 152*t*–153*t*
Diabetes mellitus
and coronary heart disease, 97, 99, 133–134
and excessive fat mass at waist, 33
obesity and, 38
research outcomes on, 119–123

Diastolic blood pressure, 46
Diet, 11, 178
and cancer, 113
combined with exercise, 39
and coronary heart disease, 97–99
and diabetes mellitus, 121–122
and muscular strength reduction, 22
research outcomes on, 40*t*–41*t*, 43*t*–45*t*
Disease prevention/management, 9*t*, 10, 95–135. *See also specific diseases*
Disuse atrophy. *See* Deconditioning
"Drop-out problem," from physical activity, 22, 121–122. *See also* Adherence, to physical activity
Dual energy X-ray absorptiometry, and body composition, 32–33
Duration of training, 17, 196–197
for aerobic exercise, 17
and balance outcomes, 81
and cognitive functioning, 52
and lipid/lipoprotein profiles, 36
for muscular strength, 22, 24
and obesity outcomes, 39

Eccentric forms, of strength assessment, 22
Economic outcomes, of active living, 11–12, 189–192
Education levels, and sedentary/active living, 3
Ejection fraction, and cardiorespiratory fitness, 17
Elbow joints, flexibility in, 28
Electrocardiogram abnormalities, and coronary heart disease, 97
Electrophysiological assessment, of cognitive functioning, 51
Epidemiological research, 12
activities of daily living, 185*t*–187*t*
anxiety outcomes, 145*t*
arthritis outcomes, 111*t*–112*t*
body composition outcomes, 43*t*–45*t*
bone health/osteoporosis, 106*t*–107*t*
cancer outcomes, 116*t*–118*t*
cognitive/psychomotor outcomes, 62*t*–63*t*
coronary heart disease outcomes, 102*t*
depression outcomes, 152*t*–153*t*
falls outcomes, 87*t*–89*t*
habitual physical activity outcomes, 177*t*
life satisfaction outcomes, 166*t*
lipid/lipoprotein profile outcomes, 43*t*–45*t*
locus of control outcomes, 164*t*
mortality outcomes, 125*t*–130*t*
muscular strength outcomes, 27*t*